Same Song, Second Verse...

Same Song, Second Verse…

✦

A Breast Cancer Survivor's Uplifting Story

By Betty Toben Warden

iUniverse, Inc.
New York Lincoln Shanghai

Same Song, Second Verse…
A Breast Cancer Survivor's Uplifting Story

iUniverse, Inc.

For information address:
iUniverse, Inc.
2021 Pine Lake Road, Suite 100
Lincoln, NE 68512
www.iuniverse.com

ISBN: 0-595-28168-0

Printed in the United States of America

This book is dedicated to every woman (or man) afflicted with breast cancer—with deep appreciation for the angels who watch over us, always.

Contents

Acknowledgements

I always read the acknowledgements in other books, and sometimes they've created a whole story about the author for me. Now that I'm writing my own, I see that it is a challenging task.

First, I want to thank my "reluctant muses," Meg Goodman and Susan Smith for their insistence that I write this and for their bird-dogging to keep me working on it. Next, Maureen Riley, my Hakomi therapist who's brought me so far in finding my own path and who helped me define my life's mission: to help others through sharing my own experiences. This book is my official beginning of that mission.

My own personal angel and "bosom buddy," Sarah Stedman, who understood so clearly why I needed to write this story and how important it could be for others. Sarah's spirituality and encouragement have become a blessed constant in my life.

The readers—Shelly Soble, Rob Sullivan, Meg, Susan, Sarah, Rachel Sternberg—and Devindra, who I hadn't met, but who cried over what he read. All of these people took the time to read the very rough first draft and to give me their kind but constructive criticisms for the necessary improvements.

A great big collective thanks to those who reached out to me with their support during the toughest times—my friends, family (and cousins-by-the-dozens), clients, and business colleagues who were there and there and there for me during my ordeals with cancer, sending me cards, e-mails, stuffed animals, muffins and beautiful flowers. I wish I could mention every single name, but my brain was cloudy for a long time and I'd hate to leave any one out.

Of course, my special love as always to the memory of my dear mom, who handled what I went through better than I ever expected (showing the strength mothers have when their kids need it), and to my wonderful son, Adam, his wife Lisa, and their "yours, mine and our" kids—Angelina, Samantha and the babe, little A.

I give my deep thanks to the universe—for always bringing me what I need at the time.

ANCIENT SANSKRIT POEM
(From Kathleen's collection)

Look to this day
for it is life
the very life of life
In its brief course lie all
the realities and truths of existence
the joy of growth
the splendor of action
the glory of power
For yesterday is but a memory
And tomorrow is only a vision
But today well lived
makes every yesterday a memory of happiness
and every tomorrow a vision of hope
Look well, therefore, to this day!

Introduction

Let me introduce myself, and tell you why I'm writing yet another book on breast cancer....

I am a happy, healthy (now) survivor of *two* primary occurrences of breast cancer—once on each side. The second diagnosis came almost exactly one year after the first.

This has been a profound experience.

The first time, I suspected there was something for me to learn from the experience—but I couldn't figure out what. When it happened again, I KNEW I had some learning to do. I don't have to be hit over the head more than twice, after all. So I paid a lot more attention, kept a journal, shared my feelings, went more inward, and reached out more to help others. And I learned about accepting. Accepting what life brings, and accepting what others chose to give me. I also learned to ask for what I need.

In both occurrences, early detection pinpointed tiny, microscopic, malignant tumors. So I had only a lumpectomy (extracting the "lump" instead of removing the entire breast) on each side—and also radiation therapy after each surgery. I'm writing this because I want to share what I learned from the first experience that made it easier for me to get through the second time around. So at the end of my story, I've included some helpful tips for all concerned—the affected person, family and friends, lovers and medical professionals.

My unique therapist, Maureen—who guided my understanding of the many other parts of me after I returned to physical health—told me that with breast cancer, the right side is from giving too much, and the left side is from not receiving enough. I've thought of that often, and of the balance we need to bring to ourselves.

I do not regret having had this experience. This may sound odd, but it's true. Others have told me that although they would never ask to have cancer, the experience enriched them in countless ways. For me, it was a life-altering experience. As you read on, I think you will see what I got out of it, what I learned about myself, and how it made me more spiritual, more centered, more appreciative, and gave me a perspective on life that I'll never lose.

I am grateful for many things, much of which I'll describe in the following pages. I remind myself often that whatever I went through could have been much, much worse. I am one of the fortunate ones.

My Hebrew name is "Bracha," which means blessing. Indeed, I am blessed.

Essay Biography, Betty Warden

One of the many things I learned during my cancer experience is that it's okay—in fact, good—for me to be open about myself with others. Before that, I would never have exposed so much, especially in any professional environment. But I had an experience that changed that kind of thinking. Part of that experience included writing this essay, which goes beyond the usual "vita," or business biography, before speaking to a group of Information Technology pros. As a result, they "knew" me—and related to me—even before I stood up to speak. Here it is:

I was born in Chicago on July 14 (the French Independence Day). I've always loved my birthday and am delighted that I had a grand celebration in Paris for my most recent landmark year!

I grew up in East Rogers Park, a Chicago neighborhood where many seem to have started out, and one which I still love. Most of my family—grandparents, aunts, uncles, cousins—lived within blocks of each other.

My mom taught dancing before I came along, and my dad was an entrepreneur with his own business in men's textiles. I think I got my "showmanship" from my mom and my business spirit from my dad. Early on, Dad was fairly successful, and we lived very well in a nice house with live-in help. I enjoyed being spoiled as an only child, with 45 dolls, pretty clothes and a dog.

When I was about seven years old, my dad lost his shirt—that's why I've jokingly called myself "Algier Horatio," since I went from rich to poor. My folks split up, and mom and I went to live with my grandparents who already shared their home with my great grandfather, my great uncle, another uncle and an aunt—it reminded me of the play "You Can't Take It With You." There were constantly people around, constant activity, lots of fun around the piano, and always additional family for meals and holidays. Already an avid reader, I buried myself in books to try to find a little "privacy." A favorite was "The Secret Garden."

In those days, it was extremely unusual to have divorced parents—so I was a bit of an oddity. In order to get positive attention, I did my best to excel in both secular and religious schools. As it turned out, being one of very few girls in a religious school served me well later in the business world in terms of relating to males as peers.

Ninety-five percent of my high school classmates went to college—with us, it was WHERE to go, not whether to go. I chose a school where I could get a state scholarship, since money was scarce. After changing majors four times during the first year, I became an English major, which enabled me to get good grades for what I loved doing—reading. I changed colleges a few times, finally graduating from Roosevelt University a semester late, after working my way through school. I had no desire to teach (which I do now and really enjoy), so I got a job at the now defunct Montgomery Ward as a catalog copywriter.

I progressed rapidly through the ranks in catalog development, going as far as they allowed a young woman to go. By that time, I was a single mom with a small boy totally reliant on my support, and I desperately needed more money. This forced me to take a stand with higher management, threatening to leave if they didn't look at my work instead of my age. That was the first time I stood up for myself in business—after that, things started to happen fast.

I became one of the first four women "allowed" to work in the merchandise department. Although I missed being on the creative side, I loved being on the business end of the company. That's where the action takes place. And that's when I realized how interesting I found the world of business. It was no problem for me being the only or first woman in my progression of jobs, since I had that early religious school experience with being a gender minority.

I was the first woman in the custom fabrics buying department, Ward's first woman Loaned Executive to the United Way, the first woman who conducted a study on hard lines (trash compactors), and the first woman in the hardware department. It was getting tiresome for me to continue to prove that a woman could work like a man, when I discovered a job opening in Ward's direct marketing subsidiary. I went after that job like a dog going after a bone and got hired during the interview. After two-and-a-half years as an assistant marketing director, I was catapulted to general manager and soon after, I became their first female vice president.

With my status and visibility, I was a role model and mentor for many other young women moving through the ranks of business. I was fortunate to have a few fine mentors who believed in me and worked with me, which contributed to my success, especially since I had never had any courses in business. Ultimately, my company sent me to Northwestern University (again, the first woman they sent), where I earned my MBA.

I left the "safety" of corporate life to join another former executive in a consulting business in 1985. Since then, I've gone back to big business a few times (Marsh & McLennan as AVP, Direct Response; Foote, Cone & Belding as VP Direct and Database Marketing) for offers I couldn't refuse. I've found there are pros and cons with anything, including working for a large company compared with being self-employed.

Now, I have my own business as a consultant in Direct Marketing, and I have two part-time jobs—one at DePaul University as adjunct faculty and the other as executive director of an educational foundation.

When I first started on my own, I had to learn how to manage my finances, how to get insurance, and about the importance of a network and a strong support system. It's a good thing I learned all of that some time back, because in 1999 I was diagnosed with cancer in my right breast. Thanks to early detection, I required only outpatient surgery—although afterwards I had to have radiation treatments for six-and-a-half weeks. I had a huge struggle emotionally and physically (due to the fatigue caused by treatment), but I got through it on the upside. I was determined to get through that with minimal disruption to my life! The experience netted me a renewed love for my family and friends, who gave me their support and prayers.

About one year later, I had a second occurrence of breast cancer on the left side. This time I knew what was ahead. So I allowed people to actually give me the help they offered. I trusted in my clients' appreciation of me, and told them to expect that I'd be working less, but still needed to work. They were wonderful, too, and stuck with me until my return to health.

The birthday on Bastille Day in Paris was extra-special as it was a landmark year as well as a celebration of health! I think I have even greater energy than before—and certainly more appreciation for all the aspects of my life.

I believe in the importance of "giving back." Life (business and personal) has been pretty good to me, largely due to what others have given to me. To that end I mentor, teach, speak, and in general, make myself available if help is needed.

> *"If you are not for yourself, who will be for you*
> *But if you are yourself, alone, what are you*
> *And if not now, when?"*
>
> —*Rabbi Hillel*

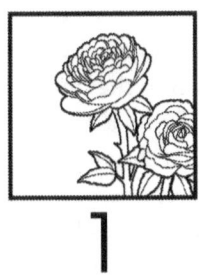

1

The Discovery

o o o o o o o o o o o o o o o o o o o o o o o o o o o o o o o o o

"Everything's got a moral if only you can find it."

—*Lewis Carroll*

I went for a routine mammogram. I am religious about doing this annually, and this time it really paid off for me, though I sure didn't feel that at the time.

After taking the film, the technician said to "hold on a minute," as the technicians always do when they go to check if the film is adequate. Usually, the technician then tells you to get dressed, although on occasion one or the other side has to be re-taken. This time, she said, "I showed this to the doctor, and I've got to take a more enlarged picture of your right side." I hummed and forced myself to be patient (not my long suit), reminding myself that I was certainly not "at risk". I told myself some minor aberration probably appeared, maybe something to do with hormonal changes.

She left with the film and returned with the doctor, a mammographer. This had never happened to me before. In the past, the only people I saw when I got a mammogram were the receptionist and the technician.

The doctor explained to me that they saw something suspicious. I remained calm, on the outside—I have a great façade I show the public. He put up my film to show me the fuzzy spots, as if I could actually see what he saw. Although I hadn't a clue what he was talking about, I nodded as if to show him I was tracking what he said. I figured that if I acted like I understood him, I'd be on "his side" and somehow everything would turn out okay.

He told me that he saw something that looked like a potential malignancy and that I'd need a biopsy to be sure. Being a businesswoman who likes to know what the deal is, I asked him point blank what could be the worst-case scenario. I always figure that if I can prepare myself for whatever is the worst possibility, I can usually handle anything that is not as bad. I even brought forth all my courage and asked him if we were talking mastectomy—to my great relief he assured me we were not. I tried to be controlled now that I'd openly addressed my deepest fear, and the doctor commented that I seemed the kind of person with whom he could be frank. (I was, briefly, very proud of the impression he had of me.) He said, of course, nothing could be sure without a pathology report—so I asked if it could be nothing, benign. He said, "Sure, that's always possible."

And then I pushed and said, "But you really think it's something, don't you?" He nodded.

I couldn't wait to get out of there.

As soon as I left the examining room I felt my head spinning. I had to re-enter the reception area to get my coat, which I put on by rote, feeling like a zombie going through motions that were possible only because of their familiarity. My thoughts were scrambled. I sensed a storm building within me as I was entering a new realm where I did not want to be, and over which I had no control.

Fortunately, the parking garage was attached to the medical building, only an elevator ride away, so I got to my car quickly.

Comfortably ensconced in the oh-so-familiar driver's seat, I just stared. This reliable car had taken me everywhere for nine years—to bring my granddaughter home from the hospital after her birth, to visit my ailing mother and run errands for her, to travel to many business appointments, to go to the cabin in the woods that I so enjoyed, to meet my out-of-town lover, and always, to bring me back home safely.

I picked up my cell phone to call someone—but who? My lover? A girlfriend? A family member? With the phone still in my hand, I burst into tears; all I could think of was Betty Rollins' book on breast cancer, "First, You Cry" and I thought—"Now I'm becoming a book title!" I could not bring myself to talk to anyone. I gathered some strength to enable me to drive home.

Somehow I arrived home safely, though I still found it difficult to place a phone call. I e-mailed my guy, desperately seeking his support (which was immediate), and then did some deep breathing before I called others. I wanted to talk with someone close to me, but I didn't know if I could. I didn't want to tell my mother or son yet…no point in worrying them before I knew anything for sure. I had no answers to any of the questions I knew they'd ask. Both of them relied on me for so much, I didn't want them to be concerned until I knew the full extent of what would lie ahead.

Finally, I calmed myself enough to phone a couple of women who've been there for me during other past trials. Although they were shocked by my news, their reactions were supportive and eventually calming, reminding me over and over that I really didn't know anything for sure yet.

I had to schedule an appointment for the biopsy. I go to a great hospital with a wonderful medical center, but the administrative support leaves something to be desired. Once I finally got through to an actual person to schedule an appointment, she said, "Is this an emergency?" I said, "Well, you tell me. I don't think I'm about to die, so it's not that kind of emergency…but if you needed a biopsy to find out if you had breast cancer, what would you think?"

She said, "I'll get you in as soon as possible!" The biopsy was scheduled for early the following week, on Thursday, November 18. (A funny thing happens when you've been hit by cancer: the key dates—biopsy, surgery, radiation—remain crystal clear for a long, long time.)

I called my gynecologist to let him know what happened and to get recommendations for a breast surgeon in case the results were positive. Thanksgiving would be soon, and I didn't want to have uncertainty hanging over my head during that long weekend. If I really did have cancer and needed surgery, I certainly did not want to wait until after the holiday to find out the details. So, being one of those overly-organized people…I figured it would be wiser to get an appointment as soon as possible and then, hopefully, cancel it if the results were benign. The secretary squeezed me in at 8:00 a.m. the Wednesday morning before Thanksgiving.

The next week seemed to take forever. I couldn't stop thinking about the "what ifs." My logic kept telling me that I shouldn't be at risk, so what could happen? No one on my mother's side of the family had been afflicted with this disease. I knew that my father's sister and her daughter had breast cancer, but I thought the paternal side didn't count as a predictor. I had a normal pregnancy, and breast-fed my son. I thought I had done everything "right"—maybe I was just worrying too much.

Respite with the Murphys

Fortunately, I already had plans to visit dear friends (the Murphy family) the weekend before the biopsy. Everyone should have friends like these people! Many years before, when Thom and Lucy first married, we had been upstairs-downstairs neighbors in a walk-up apartment building. We quickly became close. I spent a lot of time bonding with Lucy while Thom was working on his master's degree, and a lot of time with Thom when Lucy was working on her degree. So I became close with both of them, and we are now like family to each other.

Even though I was a decade older, it was the Murphys who comforted me when I had relationship-troubles, single mom troubles, a "breather" who kept calling and frightening me, problems with mice, and even seriously bad ex-husband troubles.

Thom and Lucy were always there for me, providing music, good conversation and major laughs. Even when they started their family and moved to the suburbs, I went to them for comfort when I needed huge hugs. Every time a romantic relationship got bumpy and I'd feel the need to escape, I'd run to their home for nurturing. I came to love their kids, too.

The summer before my diagnosis, the Murphys moved to another state (when Lucy accepted a professorship at a significant university). As a last hurrah and celebration of the kids' graduations from high school and grammar school, they planned a family vacation touring Europe. I wanted to go, too, so I joined up with them in Paris—but only after the whole family voted me in!

I like to think of myself as "Auntie Mame" to the Murphy kids. I encouraged both Colin and Beth to try escargot, steak tartare, wine, and finally, coffee (got Beth hooked on that)! During our trip, Beth commented to her dad, "I don't want to get old—I want to be like Betty!" They exhausted me with all the walking and stair-climbing we did (oh those Metros, those art museums), but we had a fabulous time together.

So, I went to the Murphy house the weekend before my biopsy. How could anything come out wrong when I had these dear people who loved me?

2

The Biopsy

"You're braver than you believe, and stronger than you seem, and smarter than you think."

—Christopher Robin told Pooh that last day of that golden summer...

I needed a stereotactic core needle biopsy. In spite of the fact that the procedure had been explained to me, I really didn't know what to expect. Fortunately, I had the foresight to ask my former neighbor and good friend Sandy to take me. During years of sharing a wall between our townhouses, we helped each other many times, in many ways. We were good neighbors, always being there when needed, never intruding on each other's privacy. Plus, Sandy had the added benefit of being a retired nurse and really knowing about medical procedures and vocabulary.

No matter how independent I think I am, sometimes it's just not good to go it alone. This is a lesson I keep re-learning, by the way, on both the receiving and giving ends. It's perfectly okay to ask for help and wonderful to give it.

I left Sandy in the reception area, hoping I'd see her again sooner rather than later. I left my coat and purse with her before walking with a technician, Chris, down a long hall to the room where the procedure would take place. Chris got me settled into a hospital gown and told me to climb onto the table. She busied herself adjusting the computer in front of her. Soon the doctor appeared, a tiny lady, with a medical student in tow. The doctor introduced herself and asked my permission for the student to be in attendance, which of course, I gave.

They gave me local anesthetics before I laid face down on the table which had a HOLE in it for my right breast. The doctor bent way under the table to insert a needle which would aspirate the suspicious substance. This was not a pretty picture. Anesthetics kept the area from actually hurting, but the position of my body was enormously uncomfortable, and I had to remain absolutely still for close to an hour. The doctor explained to me that two things would happen—first the extraction, then insertion of a staple. Should the results be benign, the staple would allow the area to be noted on any future, suspicious x-rays. If the results were positive, the staple would mark the spot for surgery. The doctor explained every single step before proceeding, and even showed me the needle and the tiny stainless steel staple. I felt I was in good hands.

During the procedure, the compassionate x-ray technician left the computer for a bit, and just held my left hand and stroked my arm. There were tears in my eyes—I'm not sure if they were there because I was frightened, or because of my gratitude for her kindness. Later I came to realize that although I had been holding back tears as much as possible for most of my life, from this event forward, they started to come much more easily. As a child, I tried to act very brave so people wouldn't see the hurt I felt from my father leaving. This false bravado stayed with me for much of my adult life, almost always forcing me to show a happy face whether I felt like it or not. I thought people would like me better that way.

I must have been so overwhelmed with the enormity of my situation that I just let go. Just let it all go. Now, I still cry at the drop of a hat. I have found it is not bad at all to let others know what you feel, and in fact, it is sometimes a great relief.

Since we were all women, we talked about the upcoming Thanksgiving holiday, what we were cooking, and how to prepare a turkey. Looking back, this was not only comforting, but also pretty funny. Picture this—I'm lying face down, locked in position, with one boob hanging through a hole so it could get poked and prodded, talking with a medical team about meal planning and the benefits of using a turkey roasting bag!

When I came off the table, Chris gave me an ice pack. I was glad that Sandy advised me to take caution and wear a stretchy sports bra. I just stuck that baby in there to freeze all feeling and reduce the bruising. It helped.

A few days later, the results came in positive. I kept the appointment with the breast surgeon.

My Man

Fortunately, the man in my life and I were able to get together the night before I met with the doctor. Our relationship was a complicated situation. Among other things, we lived three states apart with about 3 hours of drive time between us. We didn't see each other very frequently, and when we did, we often met in the middle. Each of us had busy schedules and many commitments, as well as established lives in our respective home towns. It took some juggling to get together on short notice, but this time we made it happen. We used e-mail and occasional phone calls for most of our communication. For some reason, e-mail seems to afford one a unique opportunity to be open and candid. I took advantage of this with him, pouring out all my feelings related to breast cancer. He was supportive and loving, telling me exactly what I needed to hear.

Once we had a plan to physically meet, we both felt almost electrically charged with anticipation and excitement, as usual. J knew how scared I was about the threat of surgery, with the fear and mystery of cancer hanging over my head. And I had the bruises from the biopsy to remind me.

We met at a comfortable motel equidistant between our homes. I got there early and made the room cozy by softening the lighting and adding candles, music, and wine. As soon as he arrived, I clung to him, feeling safe in his arms. And then we talked. J always provided for me an avenue in which I could speak my mind, without his being judgmental or argumentative. Often he gave me another perspective or new insights.

This time, I shared my deepest concerns. I knew I was only having a lumpectomy, but I feared that once they opened my breast, they'd find more.

Now, I don't have a particularly good body, but I did have nice breasts—and J loved them. I loved them, too. No matter how fat or dumpy I felt—or even when I felt particularly good—I had great tits! I used to be called a "sweater girl." Men always liked my full breasts, and teased me affectionately about them, wanting to look and hoping to touch, whether or not they did. I really liked that. (I had just moved to an apartment numbered 38-D, and the men in my life just hooted over that. Not one ever forgot my unit's number!)

So you can imagine my fears when I thought the worst might happen. Still, I had to let J know I would understand if this would be a problem for him.

I gathered my courage and asked the question, "What if I end up needing a mastectomy? Will that bother you?" I steeled myself for the answer, assuring him that he could be open with me. (In retrospect, that was probably akin to asking a man if he thinks you're too fat. What's the poor guy going to say anyway?)

J surprised me by responding almost angrily, "If they needed to lop off my arm, would you find me less attractive?" I was aghast that he'd even ask—of course I wouldn't! Once again, J provided me with a perspective that helped. I had never thought of anything happening to HIM. There is no physical thing that would have made him less attractive—nothing. I loved the essence of him.

As I think back on all I went through that first time, in spite of the many things that later happened between dear J and me, I remain grateful for his support and the way he continued to make me feel like a totally desirable woman. In spite of the after-effects from surgery, in spite of the after-effects from radiation, I felt wanted. I felt desired. I am blessed that I had such a very sexy and loving man in my life—especially then.

That special time with J was re-affirming. By the time we left to go in our opposite directions, I felt more secure and confident about facing the breast surgeon.

3

Meeting the Surgeon

○ ○

"This morning I threw up at a board meeting. I was sure the cat was out of the bag, but no one seemed to think anything about it; apparently it's quite common for people to throw up at board meetings."

—*Jane Wagner*

I requested a 5:00 a.m. wake up call so I could leave the motel early enough to miss rush hour traffic before my early morning appointment. I made great time driving which meant I could stop home first. I found it centering to have coffee at my own kitchen table and get a little grounded before going to meet the doctor.

I drove to an unfamiliar hospital where the surgeon had a branch office. Because of construction, it was confusing to find the entrance and parking lot, or maybe my head was just not clear. I was headed for a meeting I didn't want to have in the first place, and I didn't know what to anticipate. But finally I got there and found a big, impersonal, antiseptic building, practically empty at that early hour, before regular business hours. Creepy.

After I registered, I sat in a large reception area filled with people reading magazines waiting to be called. I felt like one of an anonymous group. I thought back to my beloved grandmother—I've found that I drift to thoughts of her when I need comfort, as I knew she always loved me, no matter what. In fact, I have a photo of her on my dresser, so I see her every single morning. Next to it is a smaller one of me as a child. My daily support!

Grandma Anna and Grandpa Harry

My grandparents raised me. Mom and I went to live with them after my parents split up. My grandmother cooked for me, did my laundry, and listened to me after school—mom worked during my after-school hours. It was my grandmother who made everything all right, every day. Every morning she made my breakfast and sent me to school. Mom slept in most mornings before she went off to teach classes during lunch hour, after school and in the evening. Grandma Anna was my "go-to" person when I came home from school. I loved the special affection that only a grandparent gives, and she loved having a grandchild around. So it worked well for us.

Our kitchen was a hub of activity and always smelled wonderful thanks to my grandmother's cooking skills. There seemed to be a constant stream of family and friends stopping by to enjoy the never-ending pot of coffee on the stove. Even the milkman would stop in and pour himself a cup! We had the whole family for Sabbath dinner every single week and larger crowds for major holidays. Needless to say, that kitchen was the heartbeat of our house.

I adored Grandpa Harry, too. He acted as my daily father figure, took me with him to work every once in a while, taught me tidbits about Judaism, taught me how to win at gin rummy, and let me use his car when I got my driver's license. When I started to date, he admonished me for wearing make-up (he said my grandmother never needed any, her cheeks were always rosy) and the late hours I kept—but he never gave me any rules and always trusted me.

My grandparents were married sixty-three years. They were a team. Due to severe arthritis in her hips, Grandma had been confined to a wheelchair for many years. She always expected that since she had more medical problems than her husband, she would die first. But that's not the way it happened. Grandpa Harry had a heart attack one night and died immediately, leaving us bereft and shocked that he was so suddenly gone.

After my grandfather died, Grandma went into a nursing home. She was not well enough to live alone, but absolutely refused to live with any of her children. Her father-in-law had lived with her and became a bed-ridden patient for the last several years of his life. She didn't want to put such a burden on anyone else. Once in the home, she started failing fast. She had a stroke and lasted only six weeks without her mate.

It upset me to see her treated like everyone else—just another faceless patient. I wanted to scream, "Hey! That's my grandmother! She's an incredibly wonderful, much loved person. She's devoted her life to her family. She's very special, not like anyone else!"

Sadly, to them, she was just one more person in a bed.

That's exactly how I felt in that waiting room. I had no identity other than being just another patient. I wanted to scream out, "I have breast cancer! ME!!!! I don't know why this happened, I don't know what's going to happen, and I'm just so very frightened…please help me!"

I got no special treatment—no one seemed to care about my anxiety level. I filled out a form, handed it back, grabbed a magazine to hide behind while I waited, and settled myself in a seat until my name was called. I felt I had this huge secret—I knew that even though I looked healthy and had no pain, there was something seriously wrong inside my body. I don't know exactly what would have helped, maybe an offer of a cup of coffee or tea—or some other small effort to make me feel someone there cared about me.

For solace, my mind drifted back to the night before, when I had the comfort of J's arms around me. Sometimes it helps to take myself to a different place in my mind. Even though my body sat in that impersonal waiting room, my mind took me to a loving situation.

Finally, my name was called. A nurse escorted me through the doorway to the examining rooms. I had my x-rays with me. For some reason, the hospital couldn't guarantee that those so-important pictures of detection would actually get from the facility where the mammograms were taken to a branch location in time for my appointment. So I had to retrieve them from one hospital and bring them to the other location myself.

Really! Wasn't it enough to deal with facing something so frightening without having to worry about obtaining and transporting the films that magnified my disease? I didn't even want to touch them! Oh well, another lesson we learn is to just let things like this go. These aggravations are truly minor, and there are far bigger things for our minds to dwell upon.

Fortunately, I found Doctor DJ to be a kind and gentle, albeit enormously busy man. He reviewed the films I brought, and showed me the affected area in my breast (I still couldn't exactly see it) before he explained the procedure to come. He spoke softly to me, explaining what would happen, using terms I didn't really understand. I was too nervous to ask many questions—or maybe just too nervous to even realize what I wanted to know.

The doctor assured me that the prognosis was excellent and said "…if you are going to have cancer, this is the best scenario." Yes, that's good news of course, but it's still the Big C and when it happens to YOU, no scenario sounds good. Later, I realized how really fortunate I was. Really.

I explained that being self-employed, I couldn't afford much "down" time, so we set the date of surgery for December 23, about a month away, which would give me holiday time to recuperate.

After seeing the doctor, I met privately with his nurse, Carole. She went into further detail, and also told me what I had to do to get prepared for surgery. She tried to explain the terms I didn't understand, as well as what to expect and how to care for myself. It can be very difficult to reach a busy surgeon with all the niggling questions that arise—but Carole was accessible. She became one of the many angels who cared for me.

I had to stop taking any aspirin, garlic, gingko biloba, and ginseng. Nothing that would increase blood circulation was allowed before surgery in order to prevent unnecessary bleeding. Additionally, I had to stop hormone replacement therapy ASAP.

Going off estrogen concerned me, as I thought of it as my "fountain of youth." I was told to be on the alert for bleeding, hot flashes, sleeplessness—but although I worried about it all, nothing happened. Nothing.

Oddly enough, even though this terrifying thing had been discovered, everything else seemed to go along as before.

When something devastating happens like the death of a loved one, the loss of a lover, the loss of a job—something that changes your life forever—what seems strange is that the rest of the world continues to go about its business. I reflected on this, of course, and thought here I am, worrying and worrying, when everything around me keeps going on as if nothing has changed.

My close cousin Francee lived near the surgeon's office, so I looked forward to meeting her for breakfast afterwards. She's one of my safe harbors for sharing, a special person in my life with whom I can be open and drop any façade.

I've found that what works well for me is planning something nice after I know I have to do something not-so-nice, building in a treat to look forward to instead of dwelling on dread. Sort of like when my mom took me for a hot fudge sundae after going to the dentist!

Francee and I enjoyed a sumptuous breakfast and good conversation, and I returned home to work for a couple of hours before shopping for Thanksgiving dinner. Although I was speeding inside from apprehension, I thought I was together enough—as I always have been—to get on with the business at hand. I checked my voice mail and calmly returned client calls before gathering my resources to hit the store and throw myself into meal preparation.

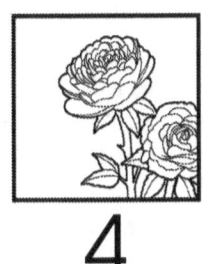

4

Thanksgiving,
or "Isn't it Upside Down?"

○ ○

"Panic is not an effective, long-term organizing strategy"

—*Starhawk*

For some reason, that year I chose to make every single dish myself. I guess I needed to keep as busy as possible…the old "busy hands are happy hands" saying came to life. I started cooking at 9 a.m. on Thursday, beginning with a favorite but time-consuming dish, ratatouille. I then moved on to the traditional turkey stuffing, sweet potatoes, green bean casserole, pumpkin pie and so on. I was so proud of myself, preparing all the food as if everything was all right. I wanted to push away the fact that in one month, my breast would be exposed on an operating table. I wanted to act and feel as if nothing had changed, when in fact, everything had changed. My whole world felt different.

I couldn't help but think of the month I had before surgery. On one hand, it seemed ample time for me to prepare myself and clear up some projects, yet on the other hand, it loomed in front of me, simultaneously seeming far off and too close. My emotions were confused, and when I allowed myself to think about this thing that grew inside me that had to be removed, I just felt dazed.

Still, I greeted my company with the best version of a radiant smile that I could muster. As usual, we grouped in the kitchen, tasting, snacking and sipping wine. I was totally impressed with myself and my competence at cooking while carrying the secret knowledge that I had cancer and needed breast surgery. From time to time, I opened the oven to check on the big bird which, to my displeasure, seemed to be cooking much too slowly.

I had an old stove, and I began to get concerned about its effectiveness. Years before I used to have friends over for an annual day-after-Thanksgiving turkey. This event began in the afternoon and lasted through evening. After we ate, we'd lounge around and watch Christmas videos to get us in the mood for the upcoming holidays. I think it all started because someone in the group got a free turkey every year, and since we all went to family functions on Thanksgiving Day, we opted to have another turkey the next day, for friends only. This became a tradition until the year my stove broke. Since I worked long hours, I rarely took time to use the oven. I didn't know it wasn't functioning until the turkey didn't cook—at all. Fortunately, my neighbor Sandy's stove worked, so we lugged the turkey over to her house. By the time dinner was finally ready, we had huge appetites, as well as a good story to tell for years to come.

I thought I was about to experience another old stove situation—only this time, without a convenient neighbor to save the day. One of my guests, starting to get quite hungry, took a look at the turkey himself and said, "Isn't it upside down?"

Yes, indeed!

So much for competence. So much for feeling cocky about how together I was. I've made dozens of turkeys over the years, and each has always come out beautifully (well, except for the time with the broken-oven). This year, my mind was clearly off in the ozone.

I chose to keep the news about breast cancer to myself. We all had plenty to be thankful for, and I didn't want to ruin anyone else's enjoyment of the meal ahead. I decided to keep quiet about myself until another time.

Needless to say, we ate late that day, but waiting for the food gave us more time to enjoy being together, sampling the appetizers and enjoying a little more wine. Once we finally sat down, we had a lovely meal and of course, the appetites were quite healthy from waiting so long!

Over the weekend, I told my mom and son about my situation. I braced myself so I could tell them, calmly, what was in store for me. I prefaced it with the good news of my excellent prognosis, told them I wasn't going to die or anything, and told them how minor the surgery would be. I wanted to downplay this difficult news so they wouldn't be overly worried. In retrospect, I'm not sure if I did that more for them or for me.

5

Before Surgery Number One

I keep saying I am blessed, and the events around my surgery proved that again.

Fortunately, I was able to see J once again that December—an "anniversary" of sorts for us. We fell in love many years back, when we were kids in our twenties, and since then our lives had taken different directions. Now, we each had established homes, family, friends and jobs in different states. More than 15 years had gone by without our seeing each other at all. We unexpectedly re-connected two years earlier and were both surprised to find there was still passion and excitement and solace. December was the month we began meeting again as we could, often at the geographic halfway point.

It was important for me to see him before surgery. I didn't know how I'd be afterwards, and I wanted just one more time when I was still "whole," so to speak. J has a scientific mind. It made him curious about cancer, and very frank and candid with his questions. I found it refreshing that he approached this with objectivity instead of just sympathetic emotion as did most others. He accepted the fact of my cancer as something that just happened to me—not anything that would alter who I was to him.

Not once at any time during the whole process did he do or say anything that made me feel less of a woman. In fact, he made me feel cherished. I carried this in my heart with me when I went in to the hospital a few days later. It helped.

I tried to cram in a lot before the date of surgery—not the least of which was getting all the holiday shopping and gift wrapping out of the way, as well as finishing up work assignments, cleaning my house, doing the laundry, etc. Even though I was told recuperation would be quick, I didn't believe that one bit!

I completed all my pre-surgery preparations, which greatly pleased my anal retentive side, when Nurse Carole called. She apologized as she told me that something came up, and the doctor would have to postpone surgery for one week. All my plans, foiled!!!

My apprehension renewed, as I faced an empty Christmas weekend. Of course, I convinced myself that the cancer would grow exponentially in that additional week, and worse yet, my plans had to be changed! Now I'd be facing a December 30 surgery date, absolutely ruining my hopes of a big welcome for the year 2000. And who knew how I'd be, physically, the first week of the New Year when I had so many work plans and classes to teach?

I hated the fact that Dr. DJ, who seemed so kind and understanding when we met in his office, could seem to be so cavalier about pushing back the date of surgery. My head was set for December 23. I scheduled my life around that date. I had plans, for goodness sake!

Granted, being a Jewess, Christmas means nothing to me from a religious perspective. But I do love the spirit of giving during that time, and gladly partake in it. Even my religious grandfather was interested in Christmas. He found watching midnight mass on television fascinating, telling me how similar it was to Jewish services of those times…replete with the swaying of incense, originally used to offset the body smell of crowds in times when there was no convenient bathing, but now used only for tradition.

I spent Christmas morning with my darling granddaughter, Angie. Always my joy. Afterward, I phoned my special friends, Kathleen and Steve. Just one month before my own diagnosis, Kathleen had been diagnosed with stage IV colon cancer. We felt a sort of "sisterhood" with a horrible bond, so I really wanted to see her.

The story about Kathleen follows, but suffice it to say, the Christmas I spent with her was most memorable—the most meaningful Christmas I have spent with anyone.

6

About Kathleen

○ ○

"Life is no brief candle to me. It is sort of a splendid torch which I have got a hold of for the moment, and I want to make it burn as brightly as possible before handing it on to future generations."

—George Bernard Shaw

Ahhhh, Kathleen, who became so dear to me, before we lost her...

I'd become quite friendly with a colleague, Steve, and got to know his wife, Kathleen, through social events and occasional travel together. Steve headed the department at the university where I taught on a part-time basis. He and I really enjoyed working together as well as getting to know each other on a personal level. Frankly, I felt closer to Steve than Kathleen—until cancer struck our lives.

In October, Steve and I were at an annual conference out of town, when he told me he had to cancel our dinner plans and return home. His wife, Kathleen, had been coughing and tired for weeks. She needed to go to the hospital for all kinds of explorative testing and asked Steve to come home right away.

The results of those tests were terrifying: stage IV colon cancer. Immediately, their lives changed with the unwelcome addition of panic and doctors and treatments and medications. From all of this—and there was so very much—a "new" Kathleen emerged.

17

The Kathleen I met originally was nice, rather reserved, certainly intelligent (she had been a French scholar, then a librarian), and reasonably sociable. The Kathleen that emerged proved to be independent, strong in voicing her beliefs, and forthright, with a candor that I found both refreshing and surprising.

My own diagnosis came one month after Kathleen's. Although mine was only stage zero—the earliest stage—cancer is cancer, and it caused a bond between us that still brings tears to my eyes, even years later.

I hesitated to tell Steve about my diagnosis, knowing that he and Kathleen were scared themselves, dealing with a potentially terminal situation. But we were friends, and I didn't want to hold back this kind of information. Besides, I worked for him, and he needed to know that I might not be functioning at my usual level for a while.

Once the news was out, both he and Kathleen got on the phone and called. They lived a long drive from me, but I promised to try to get there to visit with her. Steve spent all his time with her, of course, and I thought they could use a different face to look at. As it turned out, Christmas day presented itself as the best day for a visit.

We decided that since I wouldn't be spending the holiday recuperating as originally expected, that time could be an opportunity to visit, if Kathleen had the energy. I felt blessed that my surgery had been postponed, so I could spend that day with her and Steve. This was yet another occasion when I believed the universe moved for me; that the opening of my calendar for that day was more than a coincidence of re-scheduling.

Our plans were for me to call them in the morning and see how Kathleen was feeling, first. If she was up to it, I'd come out—but only for a short time as she tired very easily. If she wasn't up to it, I'd stay home.

When I called, Steve was hesitant, but Kathleen felt strongly about my coming to visit. I assured him that I'd plan to stay no more than an hour and that I'd leave the minute he gave me a signal.

Are you surprised to hear I had the most memorable Christmas ever and that I stayed the entire afternoon? We talked and talked. Steve served tomato soup and sandwiches for lunch. For dessert we enjoyed a coffeecake that their daughter had brought them for Thanksgiving, before returning to her job in Germany. We had a lovely time. The phone kept ringing and ringing, so I'd talk with Steve when Kathleen was on the phone and with Kathleen during Steve's turn on the phone. Both of them seemed relieved to have someone with whom they could speak openly.

What I found was a Kathleen who talked with total candor, who shared her wishes, who was anxious to talk about herself and her life, and how she wanted to live as fully as possible for whatever time she had left. She wanted to travel while she could (which they did) and spend as much time with Steve as she could (which they also did).

They had just returned from a visit to the West Coast, where Steve's brother had just re-married. He lost his first wife a few years earlier and had found a new love. Needless to say, this was an extremely emotional situation for Kathleen, but she handled it beautifully, even finding a way to comfort her niece who had difficulty accepting her father's re-marriage.

Kathleen told me she wanted to make a video about herself, so her unborn grandchildren would get to know a bit about her and her family. The woman who seemed an introvert before, wanted to see all her family and friends—everyone dear to her. I asked her if she wanted a big party to see everyone, and she replied resoundingly, "YES!" Steve was on the phone when she said that to me, and when he handed the phone over to Kathleen, I shared the party idea with him. He couldn't believe it, since his wife had never liked that sort of thing before. But things can change when mortality is breathing down our necks!

Kathleen told me that although she had always loved reading and hearing the news, she no longer had an interest in the newspaper or TV. Her own life took precedent. Both she and Steve had become interested in nutrition, as had I, so we shared information about foods and supplements and books on healthy eating. Later, I sent her a care package that included soy nuts. I wanted to do something tangible.

Kathleen had the consideration to ask if I wanted them to call me after my surgery. I told her I preferred e-mail. She understood completely that I wanted to minimize phone conversations.

What really happened that day? Kathleen and I opened up to each other as never before. We had the bond of cancer, ugly as that is. I felt privileged that she shared so much with me. Maybe this happened because both of us knew (inside) that her situation was terminal, and we didn't want to waste the treasure of our time together on small talk.

I hope I helped Kathleen in providing her a forum to speak candidly. Later, she helped me, and continued to do so even after she passed on.

We kept in touch by phone for the months that followed. During that time, I spent my own six-and-a-half weeks in radiation, which made me too tired to make the long drive to see her. At one point, Kathleen intervened for me with Steve when I told her about the poor job I did on grading due to brain fog. She understood my situation exactly, since her head had fogged up too, and she had trouble balancing checkbooks. So it was she who explained to her husband (the head of my department) that I wasn't just "tired," and that he simply had to find a way to let me revise the grades. He did just that, and I felt a lot better that my students didn't have to suffer just because I was having a tough time thinking clearly.

To my delight, Kathleen looked radiant at her birthday party that spring. I was tired from radiation treatments at the time, but I wouldn't have missed that event for anything. Kathleen had lost weight, yes, and she had less hair—cut very short and quite fashionably. She looked terrific! People packed the house that night, dressed up and pretty and chatting and cheerful. It was a grand time!

It wasn't until months later in the summer that I next saw Kathleen. I kept tabs on her progress through Steve (and his assistant, Juliet) and knew about all the times in and out of the hospital, about her trials with chemotherapy, and about her weakened state. Finally, I drove out to visit Kathleen with Nina, another professor-friend who worked with Steve and me.

Steve had introduced me to Nina some time back, and we liked each other immediately, but never really took the time to get to know each other better. I really appreciated having company that day and got a big bonus when Nina and I sort of "bonded" during the ride. (It's amazing what two women will tell each other in the confines of a car during a long drive!) That turned out to be an especially good thing, because we needed each other's comfort on the way home.

I thought it would be nice if we brought an assortment of ice cream and sorbet. For some reason, I could almost feel the metallic taste I imagined Kathleen had in her mouth (which she admitted she did indeed have). She had been through several surgeries (the cancer had spread) and treatments and drugs, and was now going through radiation.

When we arrived at the house, Steve came out to greet us and warn us of what to expect. Still, I wasn't prepared for the tiny, curled-up person I saw in that hospital bed residing in the family room. The very room in which we sat and talked so comfortably just the prior Christmas was now a place of medicine bottles, supplies and equipment. Kathleen suffered terribly from the ravages of the disease and the effects of chemotherapy.

Yet, when I walked in, she greeted me with a welcoming, "Oh, Betty!" Need I tell you how my heart warmed to hear that almost as much as it hurt to see her?

We all shared the assorted cartons of Ben & Jerry's delights. Kathleen even managed a few bites that Steve fed her. She liked the orange sorbet best. Thanks to my woman's intuition, I knew she would.

We talked about how she felt—everything hurt her, she was miserable. She told us how much additional pain she experienced getting into the car to go to radiation therapy. And then she looked at me and said, "You did it, Betty—so I can, too!" Nothing has humbled me more.

Kathleen gave me so much when she opened up to me early on, helping me realize the importance of verbalizing and sharing feelings—with loved ones, with close friends, and especially with someone with whom there is a common bond.

In August, not even a year after her horrible diagnosis, Kathleen lost her battle. Her daughter lovingly gathered some of her mother's writings and favored quotations and had copies made as a memorial. The words were a tribute. I kept them in my journal and read them many times later, which is how Kathleen helped me the second time I had cancer. I've included them at the end of this book, in hopes that this eclectic collection of hers will continue to help others.

7

The First Surgery—Where did They Think I was?

○ ○
"Pain is inevitable, suffering is optional."

—Unknown

My dear friend, Lucy, stayed with me for a couple of days before the big event. She is the most upbeat, productive, energetic woman I know and like a sister to me. Since we had been neighbors before her kids were born, it feels like we've lived together. Lucy kept me active—taking me to movies and restaurants and shopping and all-purpose running around and fun stuff. Anything to take my mind off me. Or rather, off my breast.

She insisted on prolonging her visit to take me to the hospital the day of surgery, December 30.

First, Lucy took me to the Medical Center, across the street from the hospital, because I needed to have a wire (yes—a WIRE) inserted into my right breast, pinpointing the spot of the tumor that had to be removed. Since the hospital was still in its seemingly ever-lasting period of construction, the covered overpass between the medical center offices and the main hospital facility was down. That meant I had to return to the car wearing a surgical gown, with this thing sticking out from my breast, and therefore I had to get my winter jacket over it enough to keep me covered and warm.

We had to <u>drive</u> across the street. Normally, that would have been a short walk, but hospital regulations, as well as winter weather, forbade that. So Lucy drove us to the front door and gave the car to a valet. Phew! I certainly did not want to wait in that lobby, semi-dressed, while she parked the car herself.

Believe me—it's pretty intimidating to enter a huge hospital with all kinds of people scurrying purposefully about when you don't know where you're going and you have your guard totally down. Translation: undressed! It felt very strange to be in my weird winter pre-surgical "costume," walking around with Lucy while we looked for the out-patient section of the hospital, consciously trying to avoid the eyes of normally-dressed hospital visitors and workers.

Finally, we got there—and of course, they were expecting me. In fact, they were waiting for me, wondering where I had been. The lack of communication amazed me. It was not MY idea to get a wire inserted in my breast before coming there. Where did they THINK I was? Couldn't they have called to check on me? This did not elevate my confidence.

A nurse escorted me to a pleasant, private, outpatient room. It had no bed, just a recliner chair, closet, bathroom, and stuff like that. Nothing in that room made me feel like anything bad would happen.

Another nurse came in and told me to undress before she took my vitals. She talked to me, explained the procedures, and put stretchy white leggings on me. Quite soon the gurney came to wheel me away, and I waved goodbye to Lucy. Since Lucy lives in Ohio and planned to drive back that day, she planned to hand me off to my cousin Francee who would arrive a little later. Once they knew I was OK, Lucy would leave and Francee would take over. She'd take me home as soon as I could get myself up and walking. Teamwork. It's all about teamwork.

As soon as the gurney pushed through the pre-surgical doors, an entire team of people surrounded me, poking and prodding and asking questions. At least four times one team member or another asked if I was allergic to anything. Finally, I asked them why they didn't talk to each other about my answers, instead of my repeating the same thing over and over. But everyone was very nice, very reassuring, and then Dr. DJ appeared with his gorgeous blue eyes, wearing a sports jacket. I don't know why I remember that, but I do recall thinking he looked so "casual" compared to the medically-outfitted team around me. For some reason, I found it comforting that my surgeon was dressed in street clothes, though he assured me he'd soon change. It was a touch of familiar reality in the midst of all the identical, antiseptic, surgical uniforms.

The anesthesiologist hooked me up to his magic potions, and I barely remember counting backwards. I have no memory at all of being in the surgery room. The next thing I recall was returning to the outpatient room and being helped into that comfy recliner. About two minutes later the door opened and Francee appeared with a big smile, so I knew all was well. Thanks to drugs, at that point I felt pretty okay.

Francee took me home as soon as we were excused. She stayed with me until I took a painkiller. As I began to nod off, she had the good grace to leave so I could sleep and sleep. She knows me well enough to know that sleep does wonders for me when I don't feel well. As the drug filters wore off, I started to feel like I had been hit by a truck.

With the help of painkillers and ice packs, I got through the night on my own. I felt weird when I woke up in the morning. I noticed slight pain and some discomfort which was partly physical and partly remembering that I had just been operated on for cancer. I knew there was a chance that I'd need radiation, depending on the results of the biopsy taken during surgery. I hoped against hope that the tumor remained a tiny thing and that I would require no further treatment.

Later that day Amy came to visit and care for me, but by then I was waiting on HER. I think I took all of two pain pills the entire day, although I did rely heavily on ice packs—and I had to sleep on my left side (my favorite, anyway). It was December 31, so Amy invited a friend to join us and celebrate. He brought some wonderful goodies to eat and drink before the three of us went to a neighbor's for a New Years Eve party. Amazing! I managed to hang in there until about 1:30 a.m. before I needed another ice pack and more sleep. When I woke up the first day of the New Year, I hardly felt any pain at all.

The next steps were hearing about the results of the pathology report, getting the stitches out, going for a mammogram, and finding out if I needed radiation therapy. Still a lot of scary things to face, but I was relieved to start a new year cancer-free.

8

The First Month After Surgery

o o o o o o o o o o o o o o o o o o o o o o o o o o o o o o o o

"A woman watches her body uneasily, as though it were an unreliable ally in the battle for love."

—*Leonard Cohen*

Just because the operation's over, doesn't mean you're home free. Lots of medical stuff soon follows.

In all truth, the recuperation from the surgery itself was pretty mild. There are reminders, of course. Until the stitches came out, I had to take my showers backwards so I wouldn't get any water on my right breast. And of course, there's the time when the bandages would come off, and I'd have to look. But by then, everybody else has looked so much I was almost ready to see for myself.

Still, as minor as a lumpectomy can be, it is still a mutilation of sorts. The only surgery I had ever had in my life before this had been on my feet—not nearly as personal nor intimate as one's breast!

The docs keep you busy. There seems to be one thing after another—either waiting for results of tests, or appointments for more examinations, or seeing another doctor, or something else.

Because of the long New Year weekend, I had to wait longer than usual for the results of my pathology report. Finally, the doctor called and told me that instead of my original stage zero diagnosis, I had stage I, and the DCIS (ductal carcinoma in situ) turned out to be a few millimeters invasive and not totally contained after all (the invasive stuff is what can get scary). He assured me my prognosis remained excellent, and that fortunately, the margins were clear. That sounded like very good news, even though I didn't really know what it meant. What were margins, anyway? What was he telling me?

As I write this, I notice how familiar I've become with so much cancer terminology that I never wanted to be part of my vocabulary. But at that time, I hadn't the slightest clue what "margins" were! I've a pretty decent vocabulary, and my friends are pretty knowledgeable. I put the question of definition out there to my network—but this one stumped us. We knew about some type of margins, of course, like columns on the sides of a written page, and we knew about statistics which have margins of error—maybe that's what he was talking about? Not that it mattered, since the news was good, but I am intellectually curious, especially when it's about my own little self.

Additionally, he told me a breast cancer committee convened every Monday morning, and that my case would be reviewed to determine if further surgery would be advised because of the slightly invasive nature of my tumor. Later, I learned that sometimes they just don't take out enough tissue to be sure that every bit of malignancy is removed. In those cases, a second surgery has to be performed. The fact that this possibility existed added to my agitation.

Since the tumor was stage I, not stage zero after all, he told me I'd need radiation therapy, for sure, and that the committee would also determine if I'd need chemotherapy.

The following weekend, while drinking coffee and reading the Sunday newspaper, I saw an article about breast cancer. It clearly explained that the margin was the area around the tumor. A certain amount of clear, non-cancerous tissue was a good and necessary result after the removal of a malignant lump. That is when "the margins are clear."

Doctors often tend to talk in short form—using phrases and acronyms that we poor patients do not recognize. (Having gone through this experience twice now, I realize that one thing easier the second time around was the language itself.)

It seems every business has its own language. I've often thought that industry-specific terminology is used as an underlying way of keeping outsiders out. This seemed particularly true to me in the area of systems and computer technology where, as a client with a marketing perspective, I came to believe that those guys had their own elitist approach and just wanted to "talk amongst themselves." Eventually, I forced myself to learn enough of that jargon to be able to hold up my end of the conversation. The medical world, however, seemed much more difficult to understand. The jargon from one specialty leads to more jargon in another.

I pose this question—why aren't neophyte patients given a glossary of terms specific to our type of cancer? In the first place, we are scared and very likely not thinking clearly. We are entering an unfamiliar area that will take over our lives, and the professionals in that area communicate to us with a whole new vocabulary. This can be very confusing until we sort it out. That's why I've included a glossary covering terms that I experienced at the back of this book.

To my huge relief, the breast cancer committee decided that I did not need more surgery or chemotherapy.

Medical visits kept me busy during that January. First, I had to visit my regular internist on January 4, and then on January 14, the breast surgeon removed my stitches. Right after that I met with the radiation oncologist, a wonderful man. Dr. Bill seemed truly interested in my life and responsibilities; he asked about my work, about the book in my hand and what I liked to read, and he especially wanted to know about the classes I was teaching.

I shared with him my concerns about being self-employed with no back-up and no billings unless I worked. I told him how I worried about getting everything done while undergoing radiation treatment every single day for six-and-a-half weeks.

He was totally understanding—and kind. Dr. Bill assured me that radiation wouldn't begin until a month after surgery, since my poor breast had to heal before I started the treatment. That gave me a thirty-day window of opportunity to schedule all my meetings, as well as the possibility of working ahead of deadlines for my clients.

On January 21 I had a right-side mammogram. This was painful for my still-tender breast, but the considerate technician understood that and worked as quickly as she could. I needed—and received—an "all clear" before beginning treatment.

Boob-in-a-box

My primary interest was finding out what time my daily (Monday through Friday) appointments would be, so I could work my life around that schedule. I still had no intention of dropping any balls, and to that end, I needed to carefully schedule my activities. However, the appointment time is the last thing they tell you.

At first, I was crazed at what seemed to be a lack of urgency about setting my daily time for therapy. Later I realized that because so many people are coming and going out of treatments of different duration, the only way for them to schedule is right before each new person begins. Plus, they couldn't be more helpful in trying to make it as convenient as possible for the patients.

Before radiation starts, the patient has to endure a long session of being absolutely still. During this "simulation," measurements are taken and calibrations are calculated so that the radiation rays hit the exact spot with precisely the right amount of rads every single one of the 33 times they're going to hit you. Additionally, a form is custom-molded to hold your body and head in exactly the same position every single time.

The simulation caused the worst pain I endured throughout this whole experience. Nothing invasive happened, but I had to keep my right arm elevated for about 45 minutes with no support at all. Finally, what little muscle I have started to tremble until I could no longer control that part of my body. It was like a palsy. I suffered uncontrollable arm shaking. They gave me a break for a few minutes to rest. Then we went right back to it with me, in agony, holding my arm up straight until finally they finished. Once that part was over, I relaxed my arm and shook it out.

Next came the markings. To my surprise, "x's" and lines connecting them were drawn on my body with a black, felt tip pen, making sort of a box around my right breast. Little pieces of transparent tape (yes, the kind you use to wrap packages!) were placed over the "x"s to protect them. The doctor told me to take extra special care when bathing, so the markings would remain for my first treatment. At first, it was very depressing and a bit frightening to see my body mapped with a felt tip pen. Later, when my sense of humor returned, I referred to this as my "boob-in-a-box."

The experience made me feel like a little helpless person in a large room all by myself, with big equipment over me. The doctor and technician isolated themselves by entering into a glassed-in cubicle. Waves of feeling so very alone kept washing over me.

Little did I know that I'd feel even smaller when I started the actual radiation treatment.

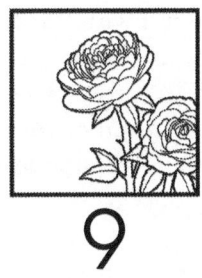

9

The First Radiation Treatment

"A book is a garden carried in the pocket."

—Chinese Proverb

The first treatment was at 11:15 a.m. on Friday, Jan. 27—about one month after surgery. New patients are taken only between certain hours (in this case, between 11:00 a.m. and 1:00 p.m.), so the doctor and the team can spend more time with you than they do with those already in the routine of regular, daily treatments.

Here's what happened.

First, I had to check in with Nuclear Medicine reception. To begin with, entering a room that says "Nuclear Medicine" feels weird. It made me expect to come out glowing with a strange, reddish, luminescence.

Next, I went to the waiting room, where there were plenty of chairs, some magazines and a television. I'm the type of person that prefers to go inward when I'm in a new situation (I've often said I'm a closet introvert) and also the type who brings a book everywhere. I just wanted to escape into whatever I was reading until my name was called. I did not want to talk to anyone. I did not want to watch TV. I did not want to be there.

I tried not to think of anything other than the book I had with me. I could not imagine what was waiting for me and did not want to think about it. I figured I'd find out soon enough. In retrospect, I wish I had brought someone with me. Too many of us go through these experiences more alone than necessary.

Nicely, when your name is called, it's by a cheerful technician who comes to personally escort you into an entire suite, containing another smaller waiting area, a large reception/work area, a medical scale, the huge radiation room, and a rabbit warren of offices, examining rooms, changing rooms, and bathrooms. Now the fun begins.

I was taken to a changing room, given a hospital gown and told to strip to the waist. The head-high mirror in the room meant I could barely see my affected breast—not that I wanted to look.

Once I changed into the gown, the technician escorted me to the radiation room. This was truly intimidating. A giant semi-circle of very serious-looking equipment hovered over a narrow table. My custom-molded form sat on the table waiting for me, identified by the last 4 digits of my social security number. I had to remove my hospital gown and, naked to the waist, climb up on to the table and then lie down, placing my back and neck to fit precisely into the molded form. Exposing my entire upper body added to my feelings of vulnerability. As soon as I positioned myself, I was introduced to the team. Kids! Sweet young women and yes, even one guy. At first the presence of a male made me uncomfortable, but it soon made no difference.

They explained what would happen. The machine and the table would be set at exactly the same positions for every treatment. The table would be raised, electronically, to be better situated under the giant machine, which would rotate around me until its nozzle would point at the precise location on my breast every time. No one actually said I'd be "zapped," but that word worked for me. They told me how long it would take (maybe a minute) and that they'd be out of the room, on the other side of the wall, monitoring, watching and listening by video. So I could talk to them if I wanted. Even though this is all carefully explained, there is nothing in my life that prepared me for the totally vulnerable feeling I experienced once I was left alone, lying under that huge apparatus on a narrow table too high off the floor to escape on my own. I felt abandoned. Terrified. I imagined falling off. I wanted to cover my exposed breasts. I wanted to tell them to stop. I did NOT want to be radiated.

But I had no choice.

Radiation continued for 32 more treatments.

10

Daily Treatments

○ ○

"When people talk, listen completely. Most people never listen."

—Ernest Hemingway

I started my daily radiation treatments with no small apprehension. In the first place, since becoming self-employed I'd come to resent any fixed daily schedule and secondly, this wasn't a routine I looked forward to. I reflected on this that first Monday, as I drove to a 4:15 p.m. appointment that I would have to keep every single weekday for the following six weeks.

The doctor told me that at first, I would feel nothing, and that the effects would be cumulative. This became a reality all too soon. After the first couple of weeks, I felt great on Sundays and for the beginning of the week. By the end of the week, through Saturdays, I felt tired. Tired? No, actually fatigued. Overwhelmingly exhausted.

I found myself unexpectedly glad that my adult son was living with me and home from work about the time I returned from the hospital. I liked having him there.

Adam

I had been a single mom most of Adam's life and raised him with little help. He was a darling baby and loved to cuddle. When I'd hold him, he'd put his head in my neck and just drop his arms, totally secure that I would not let go. And I never did.

We struggled terribly—especially financially—during the early years. Once, I had just ten dollars until my next paycheck, until my long-time friend Rachel drove an hour across the city to give me enough money to get by until the next payday. Another time, I spent my entire savings, one hundred dollars, on an old car so I could get Adam to day care. "Old Blue" had no heater and only the driver's door would open and close, but it was reliable and much easier than carrying a small child and diaper bag, standing on street corners waiting for public transportation. The carburetor would stick every once in a while, so I carried a special rock in the trunk that I used to hit just the right spot—this really impressed a couple of mechanics. Plus, it had a great Stromberg-Carlson radio. I loved that car!

By the time my son hit adolescence, my financial situation improved enough to enable me to buy a home. I chose a charming townhouse with three bedrooms, two baths, a full basement and a cozy fireplace. There was plenty of space for both of us and the friends and family who often came to visit.

It took a year of house-hunting, but it felt right the first time I saw it. That little house exemplified my father's fine advice about home selection: "Your home should make you feel that it welcomes you and holds you in its arms."

Adam was not an easy kid to raise. Although he always had the sweet core that emerged so clearly in maturity, it was often difficult to find during those teen years. Adam was a handful, with a temper that periodically erupted, sometimes at the least provocation. I lived with a constant stream of large boy/men tromping up and down the stairs, a constant beat of heavy metal emanating from Adam's room, a barrage of phone calls, and an ever-emptying pantry.

This lasted much longer than I anticipated. I always thought I'd just have to hang in there until he became eighteen and went to college. But life didn't work out that way, and Adam didn't move out until he was twenty-five. Finally, I had some peace and quiet.

Nothing is more welcome to an avid reader like me!

I had always told my son, "No boomerangs. Once you're out, you're out!" But resolve weakens all too often with one's child—no matter how old that child may be. Unfortunately—well, ultimately, not *really* unfortunately because things worked out wonderfully for Adam years later—a divorce caused my son to become a single dad. Adam moved back into the townhouse, temporarily, and on weekends his daughter Angie joined us.

This was a difficult time in my life. I became very depressed when my new-found freedom ended, my job wasn't going well, and my romantic relationship wasn't working. I was also taking diet pills (yes, Phen-fen) and hormone replacement therapy, and either that combination, or the unhappiness with my life, plunged me into the worst depression I've ever experienced. I was borderline suicidal. Thanks to the persistence of dear ones—cousin Francee who talked to me nightly, and girlfriend Lucy who pushed me to seek help. At her insistence, I called my doctor for an appointment to discuss my medications, and I looked for a therapist. Finding a good therapist is a gift, and I was blessed to find Maureen. Our weekly visits became the highlight of my life.

Finally, Adam found his own place to live, and I returned to the joys of my privacy.

Soon after, I decided that since I lived in a city situated on a huge, beautiful lake, which I loved—especially being a Cancerian (interesting astrological nomenclature, eh?)—I had no reason not to be closer to the water. I wanted to more easily enjoy its soothing qualities and its magnificence. So I started looking around for a new home.

The problems with most of the places I saw were not enough space for my books, not enough storage, no place for a home office, or no parking. Then I found a two-bedroom, two bath condo practically sitting on my beloved Lake Michigan. It was spacious, light, airy and affordable. The views from every window were astounding! The huge master bedroom would be for me, the other would serve as a home office/guest room—or a "hoffice," as the trend expert Faith Popcorn calls it. I kept pinching myself at the thought that I would be living there. I sold the townhouse for the same amount as I paid for the condo. Just too good to be true, I thought, as I moved there in early fall, 1996. I felt so good to be there, I even stopped seeing my therapist.

Never did I imagine that my son would join me!

But that's what happened. Over Labor Day weekend in 1999, my dear son lost his home due to an ugly separation from his female roommate and came to stay with me, temporarily. That "temporary" situation lasted close to a year. At first, we had quite an adjustment to make, since we were both used to having our own space.

As it turned out—here's where the universe moved so favorably once again—he was right there the entire time from my diagnosis through all the radiation treatments. I will never forget how important and supportive were his morning hugs, and the daily "How're ya' doing, mom? You getting through it okay?" One day, when I was particularly tired and just couldn't drag myself out of bed before he left for work, Adam came in my room and asked for my cell phone. At first I was annoyed, until I saw that he had a cell phone cover for me with a sunflower on it to cheer me up.

Every weekend my darling granddaughter, Angie, was there, too. She was about seven years old at the time, and a loving, delightful child. Nothing cheered me more than making breakfast for the three of us when sometimes with the least encouragement, we'd all break into laughter and hugs.

The most important things to me during radiation were being loved, hugged, and enjoying laughter! (Actually, those things are still important to me—but even more so, then.)

Having my son stay in my home office/guest room turned out well; he was only there after work when I was too tired to use the computer anyway. I'd come home from radiation, do something about dinner, read or stare at the TV for a bit, and then I went to bed. I was in bed a lot! My cat, Friday, was quite happy about that. Friday is a lap cat and likes to hang on me whenever he can. He was delighted to find me lying down so often and being so very available to him.

Once I found my preferred route to the hospital, the daily trip quickly became one I drove almost on auto-pilot. The waiting room also became part of the routine. The highlight was meeting Sarah, who became—and remains—my angel. She was one of the unexpected delights of the waiting room. More about Sarah (and angels) soon…

"X" Marks the Spot

At the onset of radiation, I was offered the benefit of tattoos. These are tiny permanent dots marking the affected area, placed where those "x's" had been for my felt-tip boob-box. If you refuse the tattoos, then you need to continue to have felt-tip pen markings, taking extra care to keep them intact the entire time. That means very careful showering and repeated applications of the markings all throughout the six-and-a-half weeks.

I thought the tattoos would make my life easier, but I was still vain about my cleavage and didn't want it marred. Also, my religion does not support permanent body-marking. An understanding—and brilliant!—technician had given herself a tiny pin dot between her thumb and forefinger, to show patients what the tattoos looked like. She knew that many of us would imagine them to be far more obvious than they are. Once I saw hers was no more than a mini-freckle, I agreed to them immediately. After a quick and simple process, I had my tattoos. That meant I could wash off the black, felt tip pen marks that were so ugly, and I would be freed from worrying about water damage when showering.

Later, I was even more thankful I made this decision. When I found that I needed radiation, again, on my left side, the tattoos on the right side clearly defined the previously treated area. Radiation can be administered on the same area only once; there would be too much harm a second time. Those tiny tattoos protected me from overlapping radiation rays the second time around. Another way the universe moved for me.

The folks in the waiting room candidly discussed whether or not to get tattooed. One lady nearing the end of treatment said she refused because she wanted no additional reminders of going through the ordeal of breast cancer. Even as she said it, long before I knew what a remarkable experience my having cancer would be for me, I thought I was not like her at all. I wanted to "mark" this life event. Somehow, I sensed it would be life-altering as, indeed, it was.

Still, I liked to listen to that woman. She had been through chemotherapy before radiation and covered her bare head with a special hat. It impressed me to meet someone who was almost done and who got through it all, and who appeared to be ready to return to a "normal" life. I needed the life-goes-on affirmation.

Another woman complained about everything. She had a deep tan so her skin looked sort of leathery. She groused about the daily drive to the hospital, about her exhaustion, about how badly her skin reacted to radiation—she talked and talked. Her chest, she showed us, looked reddish and had broken out in a way that looked like sun poisoning. We learned from her about the importance of skin care—and where to buy cheap camisoles!

Since radiation can burn the oh-so-tender breast skin, wearing a bra becomes increasingly difficult. Some of us well-endowed types weren't comfortable going without when in public (though once at home, those devices got ripped off ASAP). The only camisoles I had seen were pricey. I knew this was a temporary situation and didn't want to spend a lot of money on short term needs. Until that waiting room tip, I never thought of going to discount stores for underthings. I soon became a regular shopper there.

A third woman came to the waiting room "as is." Her hair was just beginning to grow back after chemo, and although she often wore knit tops, she did not wear any prosthesis to hide the fact that she had a mastectomy on one side. She stood tall, and I always thought, proud. She was alive! She knew that mattered more than anything else.

We shared tips on how to shower sideways or backwards since most of us were protecting affected areas from water, about how to prepare cornflower and baking soda to replace the underarm deodorant we were not allowed to use, and about only shaving under our arms with safer, electric razors. It was very important that we protect our skin from cuts, from harsh deodorant, from anything that might cause additional harm to the area exposed to radiation.

We shared recommendations on books to read, how to build rest periods into our work and home life schedules, and how to release ourselves from non-essential commitments. We were all colors, from all economic/social backgrounds, of all ages. But we were all "sisters" in our fight against breast cancer.

11

About Sarah

"Keep your face to the sunshine and you cannot see the shadow."

—Helen Keller

The daily radiation routine starts with registering at Nuclear Medicine reception, before sitting in the waiting room until a therapist takes you to the radiation therapy suite. Once there, you get a parking pass. That doesn't mean the parking was free—it only allowed those of us going to the Cancer Center to have convenient parking spaces. A bonus!

The waiting room is fairly large, sort of mauve-ish, with magazines and a television and plenty of upholstered chairs. A few days after I started treatment, I entered the waiting room and took my usual seat against the wall, ready to open my book and read. Standing in front of me facing the TV with her back to me was a tall, lanky, blonde woman. She was wearing a brightly colored nylon jogging suit and she was stretching—feet apart, arms way up high, first with one hand pulling at the wrist of the other and bending sideways from the waist, then reversing for the other side. I figured she was some kind of athlete.

She and I had appointments just 15 minutes apart, so quite often we were either in the waiting room together, clothed, or waiting for treatment together in our hospital smocks. Dressing in those look-alike hospital gowns is a great common denominator.

We started to talk about books we were reading and what we did in our lives, and began feeling some kind of bond almost at once. People going through radiation are very careful with each other, since so much of what we used to think was important to our dignity was removed (like being topless in front of strangers, among other things). So it takes a bit to test the ground with personal conversations.

Sarah had a sweet, southern voice and seemed open to talking and sharing. Her intelligence was immediately apparent. We shared that I was in the middle of teaching two university classes, and Sarah had been a professor herself, teaching voice at a top university. After we established our credentials, we went on to talk and talk. I often felt sort of cheated when she was called for treatment and our conversations were interrupted.

It seems we BOTH felt that way. So we planned a dinner one night at a nearby health food restaurant. Again, the conversation flowed easily. I found Sarah to be creative, spiritual and very positive. She and I were the most upbeat patients our radiation team was treating, and they were very happy to see the friendship and support that grew between us.

Over time, I found out that Sarah not only had breast cancer, as I did, but that hers required two operations, and she also had a colostomy for colon cancer. Ultimately, Sarah had 4 surgeries that year—the last to blessedly reverse her colostomy! Sarah told me that upon receiving her simultaneous diagnoses of breast and colon cancer, she crumbled. So she gave herself up to the universe, asking for help. She sensed a hand reaching down to her. Sarah got through her ordeals by putting her trust in the power of the universe, and it has never let her down. That would be impossible.

The occasional dinners continued—we especially loved going to a pancake house where Sarah, who counts every bit of nutrition that goes into her body, loved to treat herself to tons of melted butter. We enjoyed this so much, that some of the radiation team threatened to join us, as they said we were having too much fun without including them.

Was I blessed? Oh yes!!!! Who else would look forward to going to radiation? Well, I did because Sarah was there.

For the next year after our joint experience with radiation therapy, Sarah and I kept in close touch. She successfully completed her colostomy reversal, and bit by bit got back to her life—swimming, playing bridge, artistic endeavors, and becoming more and more spiritual and grateful that she survived as she did.

We met for meals occasionally, and it was delightful to see her wearing darling outfits, so different from the concealing jogging outfits she wore when we first met and for which, thank heaven, she had no more need. Sarah turned out to be quite slender and was thrilled to be able to return to the tight jeans she loves.

Always, we reminded ourselves of how incredibly fortunate we were to find each other. Both of us believed that the universe put us there, giving us exactly what we needed at the time. A bosom buddy, so to speak.

Our treatments occurred during the winter season. We found we had similar attitudes about weather. Mainly, that it's just weather and as such, it is what it is—not something to fret about. One day there was an ice-storm and both of us came in squealing about how incredibly beautiful the trees appeared. Everyone else was complaining about slow driving on slippery streets, but we, instead, had chosen to look up. The medical team said we made them all feel good—and why not? We were alive!!!!

Another time, I was delighted to hear about Sarah's experience while grocery shopping in a very affluent suburb. It had been pouring outside for days, and while standing in line, Sarah heard one deeply-tanned and bejeweled socialite-wannabe complaining about how much better and sunnier it was in Florida where she had a second home, and how tired she was of the rain. The lady went on and on and on with her complaints and all those trapped in that line were stuck listening to her.

Finally, my dear Sarah, my very proper Sarah, with her most lovely, soft, southern tones, turned to the woman who was behind her in line and said, "Excuse me, may I have just one minute of your time?"

The woman was a bit surprised. Then Sarah said, "You know, I've been through four surgeries this past year, two for colon cancer and two for breast cancer. And I've come to appreciate being alive, no matter what kind of weather is out there...so I never complain about rain or anything else. It's just not all that important." (I wasn't there when this happened, but I wouldn't be surprised if the other folks in line broke out into applause—I know I would have!)

I called Sarah immediately after receiving my second diagnosis. I knew she would understand better than anyone what I was feeling, how scared I was, and what to say to me. She was empathetic, of course, but she also reminded me about the importance of learning from this experience, which gave me something strong and positive to think about.

When I had my second surgery, Sarah was waiting for me in "our" waiting room. How perfect. Seeing her there once again made me feel everything would come out all right. A short time later, walking alongside my gurney en route to surgery she pointed to a pin on her jacket and mouthed "This is for you." I hadn't a clue what she meant.

Afterwards, when my head cleared, Sarah leaned over me. She took the pin off her jacket and put it on mine. It was the backside of a little silver angel with a golden halo. Here's Sarah's angel story:

"When I woke up from the last of my four surgeries, the colostomy reversal, I found this angel pinned to my pillow. I don't know who put it there and was not able to find out, though I asked. I believe she's a traveling angel, and I kept her as long as I needed her. She's yours for now, and you can name her whatever name you choose—the right name will come to you as it did for me…But remember, she travels, so whenever you don't need her anymore, be sure to pass her on…"

I asked why the angel faced backwards. Sarah told me it was because she was watching over my heart.

I wore that angel every day for months and months. She was a pretty little thing, and many people admired her and asked me where I got her. I happily shared the angel's story with them. Often, it brought tears to their eyes, too. When the day came, I did indeed pass that angel pin on so she could watch over someone else.

I have kept my belief in angels. They are always with me now, supporting me when I need them.

Sarah's Version

I shared what I'd written about Sarah with her. The following is her view on it:

On September 10, 1999, I received—within ten minutes of each other—the double diagnoses of breast and colon cancers. Reeling from this information, stunned almost into a complete cessation of time, I pulled the emotional mask down over my face and assured my surgeon (Dr. DJ of whom Betty speaks) that I was fine, and needed to go home to assimilate it all before talking about surgeries.

And home I went. Alone, except for the guides and angels who are always with me and have been for most of my adult life. I wandered through my beautiful lake-front apartment full of happy plants, my beautiful piano and bright sunshiny colors…touching little flowers, listening to the waves, stroking my silky cat Nadia as if from a distance, listening to the ringing in my ears, and wondering how I could possibly bear the next moment of my existence. After some time I found myself sitting on my bed, and quite from nowhere came the knowledge that I simply was not capable of DOING THIS by myself. And so I spoke out loud to the Universe and my Creator, informing them that I was putting every bit of this pain and terror into their hands, that I would do whatever I was told or shown by them was necessary, but that they simply HAD to take it all over into spiritual management. Weeping in great gasps of breath, I gave my life into cosmic keeping. And suddenly, from nowhere, came a firm, strong, soft hand taking hold of my right one, squeezing it a little, and without a single word I felt safe and free of fear. It was the single most palpable, spiritually passionate moment of my life, and the foundation upon which I am building the life with which I have subsequently been blessed.

The three surgeries which followed immediately (too closely to one another, but that is another part of the story) were full of their own struggles. At last I found myself facing the radiation treatment. Alone of course, though not in a spiritual sense; it was just that there was no other real live person to be there with or for me (not one of the advantages of single life!). As is my way, I simply addressed it in stride, and appeared at the Cancer Center for my radiation as scheduled. The colostomy, which saved my life after a vicious struggle with infection, left me wearing limited styles of clothing. And so I was in my warm-up suit, doing the stretches that I hoped would give me back full range-of-motion after losing so many lymph nodes, when I first met my wonderful angel, Betty.

I can still see every detail of the waiting room, just as every moment in radiation is etched into memory as in stone. She sat in what became "her" chair, watching me (politely, of course, she is not capable of being any other way). Bright, unusually intelligent brown eyes smiling, she introduced herself, and immediately I felt the "click" of recognizing soul-family. Laughter was one of the first things we discovered in common: great, deep, hearty, prolonged laughs composed of the joy in each of us that refused to be stilled despite the trauma that lay both ahead and behind. What a wonderful smile she has, I thought to myself, and how clearly that smile goes straight to her eyes. THAT is an authentic person. What a treat, such a discovery…and later, of course, what a heartwarming gift from the universe I discovered Betty was to my life.

We wiped out the radiation staff with our joy and laughter. They wanted to go with us on our adventures and share that connection. We took them cookies and muffins, gave them big hugs and kudos—you see, they suffer on a daily basis with every person who comes through that lab. Betty and I had it in our power to make them smile and laugh, and inhale joy when we were around. And so that is exactly what we did. All that enthusiasm filtered down to our doctors, as well, and to this day we get hugs from every physician on our teams whenever we meet.

We were a remarkable, thoughtful gift of the Universe to each other; the absolute trust we KNEW between us almost immediately was part of that gift, as was the easy openness with which we shared every part of our lives. Facing such illnesses is life-altering in every conceivable way, and we embraced our spiritual metamorphoses together with huge support and ongoing joy to this very day

◆　　　◆　　　◆

Sarah and I remain close and believe we have a special bond, in fact, a spiritual connection.

To celebrate our both being cancer-free, we attended the closing ceremonies of a 3-day walk in support of finding a cure for breast cancer. The closing ceremonies were very moving, especially the silent prayers for those who didn't make it, as well as the celebrations for those of us who did. It was emotional and teary and thrilling—there is no one I would rather have been there with than my bosom buddy...Sarah.

"Never give up, for that is just the place and time that the tide will turn."

—*Unknown*

12

Effects of Radiation

My doctors, even the dear Dr. Bill, said that I'd get tired, but they weren't sure if the tiredness was from radiation, or just from having to go to treatment every single week day, 33 times. At first, I wondered about this myself, and tried to pay extra attention to how I felt so I'd know the answer. Believe me, it was the radiation!

I'm normally a fairly high-energy person, and pride myself on my competence in the juggling and multi-tasking that has become a way of life. As a self-employed consultant, it's often necessary to handle multiple client projects, meetings, phone conferences, and so on, each with different needs and deadlines.

I'm also adjunct faculty at a major university. I had already committed to teaching two student intern classes the term that would begin right after my surgery. Usually, I only teach one class a term, but there was an overload of students and I've always found it hard to refuse almost anything if I hear "I/We need you…" Fortunately we had only two physical class meetings over the term, the rest happened over the Internet. Additionally, we scheduled one-on-one, individual meetings with each student—key to the course. With two classes, that meant about 40 meetings.

Fortunately, with the help of the good Dr. Bill, I arranged most of those meetings before the grueling daily therapy schedule began.

I had been told I'd be tired, but I never expected the full extent of what that meant. And I never accounted for the fact that my brain would clog up—either with exhaustion or just plain old fuzzy-brain syndrome. I'll never know.

But I can say that although I was immensely proud of myself to get through both classes, read all the papers, and get all the grades in on time, I was horrified at the number of challenge e-mails I got from students after class was over. Fully one-third of my classes questioned their grades. At first, I took the "teacher" position and supported my own decisions…but then, as the e-mails continued, I took a further look. Soon I realized that I simply had not been thinking clearly at all. In fact, I thought, "What WAS I thinking?"

My students were right! My poor head must have been so clouded that it kept me from making good decisions.

I now advise people going through cancer treatment to try to avoid major decisions of any kind, and if that's not possible, get someone to oversee what you're doing. It took weeks after treatment until my brain felt like its old self.

Friends help a lot. A colleague of mine, Pat, happened to be going through radiation at the same time. We met regularly to share "radiation-stories" and to give each other helpful tips for dealing with our business world. We both had the same kind of meetings and conferences to get through. We bolstered each other up for these sessions, told each other which of our out-of-town friends had hotel rooms where we could rest if stuck at an all-day conference, and encouraged each other to sit when we met in the conference exhibit hall.

Pat bought two copies of "The Breast Book" by Dr. Susan Love. Her head was so fuzzy from her own radiation treatments that she forgot to give me mine, but when she heard about my second diagnosis, she sent the book by messenger. I found it fascinating, and I recommend it for every woman, but especially for those with breast cancer.

The tiredness from therapy grew to sheer fatigue. Since the effects are cumulative, about midway through the treatment period I started to really feel zonked. Normally, I practically bound of bed. I'm a disgustingly cheerful morning person. Usually, I have coffee, read the paper, go for a walk and I am at my computer checking e-mail and starting to work about 8:00 a.m. That ceased for some time.

Unless I had an early meeting and forced myself to get going, I moved very slowly at the beginning of each day. By Thursdays, I wanted a crane to get me out of bed. And I ached. Oh, how I ached. My hips, my thighs, my lower back. I felt like I was aging at an increasingly rapid rate. I understood what the pain must have been like for my mother with her arthritic hips. I just dragged myself around for the first couple of hours—and those morning walks quickly became history. I needed to judiciously parcel out every tiny bit of energy that I had left.

It wasn't until months later, talking to another survivor, that I learned the large muscle groups are sometimes affected. By that time, my aches and pains had disappeared. Still, I felt relief that those problems had been caused by radiation and were only temporary.

Oddly, this did not happen the next time.

And then there was the skin-thing. Patients are told to take great care with the "affected side" as they call it. The burning is gradual and can become quite painful. Over time, my skin began to get bright pink and very tender—it really hurt. The medical staff gave me special care creams for my radiation sunburn. The creams were so helpful and soothing, I carried a tube with me everywhere. Often, when in a restaurant or other public place, I'd excuse myself to go to the ladies' room for a quick application. Ahhhhh, sweet relief.

The tenderness is in all the places a bra would touch—the breast itself, under the breast, the underarm. Some have it far worse than I did, although in my case, the only thing that I found reasonably comfortable was a soft, large T-shirt. I wore camisoles when I had to leave the house, and loose-fitting clothes, but I couldn't wait to get home and remove anything that touched me. I learned to sleep on my right side, which I still do. Well, actually, I sleep on both sides now. I guess my experiences with bi-lateral cancer made me an ambidextrous sleeper.

My pink skin blackened after the treatment ended. One day, getting out of the shower, I looked at my breasts with shock in the bathroom mirror. My right side was very obviously darker and smaller than the left side—the darkness was around and even under my breast, like a shadow-effect. Over the next several weeks, most of the dark skin sloughed itself off and healthy soft pink skin replaced it. The size difference, however, was not temporary.

I knew I was lucky to still have a breast at all on that side, which made me feel guilty about my vanity. But frankly, with one side so much smaller than the other, I thought it looked silly and out-of-balance. Even though I knew I was fortunate to have had early detection, microscopic tumors, and a good prognosis—I kept looking askance at my different-sized breasts!

Many times during this whole process I'd look at my breasts in the mirror. Often I'd cry with the overwhelming emotion that comes along with breast cancer. I cried before surgery, I cried when I saw the stitches, I cried during radiation, and I cried when I saw the effects. I still cry when I think back on it all. My friend, Rachel, told me to think of my tears as little, pure crystals. I tried to do that.

I have never been the kind of person who openly displayed emotion. At least, not the kind that brings on tears. I've always been guarded about that, even when alone—until this experience. To this day when tears flow freely I no longer feel the need to suppress them. They're my own little crystals of feelings.

Yes, there was plenty to gripe and groan about during treatment. But I quickly realized that I had much to celebrate, also. I had every assurance that I'd be all right. So many others went through so much more, and far too many perished from this awful disease. I was alive. I would recuperate. I was blessed.

The outpouring of support touched me. It came from current friends and family, business colleagues, as well as the new friends I made, such as Sarah, and the bonding I felt with other cancer patients.

Every day I would check e-mail to find one or more uplifting messages. And the flowers—oh, the flowers. What a huge spirit-lifter for me. I have always loved fresh flowers, but since I moved into a condo which caused me to give up my garden, I appreciated them more than ever.

The supportive cards came, too. I loved every single one, and appreciated every prayer, every good wish, and every word of comfort. I felt blessed that so many thought of me during this challenging time. I even got a card about the challenge of going through radiation, sort of a "hang in there" message. It was difficult to believe there were so many of us that a greeting card had been produced.

I gave my thanks.

My condo has a very private balcony overlooking Lake Michigan which allows me to watch the sun rise. I found myself going out there many mornings to stretch, and when it happened to be early enough, waiting for the sun to appear. Watching her crest, I'd open my robe to expose my breasts, spread my arms wide to the sky and ask for strength from the sun, giving thanks that I was able to stand there and do so.

Starting a day with such a blessing renewed me and imbued me with a source of much-needed energy that I believe only the sun herself could bestow on me.

As I'd reflect on the day before and the day to come, I became more and more impressed with what was becoming truly important to me. My perspective began crystallizing. I came to realize and appreciate the strength of the love I received from my family—particularly my son and mother—as well as the power of friendships.

I began to adjust my priorities. Much of my adult life had seen me as somewhat of a workaholic, putting my work first, working killer hours, at times to the detriment of my family and other personal relationships. Sometimes I'd resent the "intrusion" of friends or family for heaping on requests for which I just didn't have the time. Noooooo, I was a businesswoman. Work came first. That had been my motto.

How quickly that changed once cancer entered my life.

13

The Celebration(s)

"I celebrate myself, and sing myself."

—*Walt Whitman*

My radiation treatments were completed on March 15, the ides of March!

Sarah's last day was two days earlier, so we celebrated by having a healthy dinner together at a local vegetarian restaurant. She brought wonderful, home-made sweets to thank our team of technician-angels. I've learned that it's important to give thanks, in any way, and let people know how much whatever they've done matters. I chose to bring flowers on my last day, as I thought they would be cheered by looking at something pretty.

I had a few days to go without Sarah's company, so I changed my treatment time from late afternoon to morning. I just couldn't bear the idea of going at my usual time and not seeing her there anymore, even though I was delighted she could begin recuperating from her treatment.

Sarah had to face yet another surgery to reverse her colostomy—not an easy time ahead, but one I knew she would meet with great anticipation, so she could get on with her life freely. I, on the other hand, would be just plain DONE—with the exception of taking Tamoxifen for five years and keeping a schedule of quarterly doctor visits for the next two years.

I started to plan a celebratory trip over the Memorial Day holiday. I wanted to fly, I wanted to go somewhere I'd never been, I wanted to get outta' town!

The last five treatments of radiation are called "boosters." I'm not sure what goes on, but it's a double zapping just to be sure all those ugly potential cancer cells are totally dead. A slight change of routine, but by this time, I had such total trust in the team they could do just about anything they wanted to me. I don't know if those boosters were so strong they made me extra-tired, or if the cumulative effect of the prior six weeks just hit me very hard. In any case, overwhelming exhaustion consumed me.

Much to my surprise, I did not feel like my old self the first radiation-free morning, nor the next, and not for some time thereafter. There were additional emotional problems causing me strain in that my mother had been hospitalized and soon, I'd have to bring her home. She was weak and aging and could no longer live completely on her own, so I had to arrange for some kind of in-home care. Another heavy drain on my already sapped energies, but helping my mother could not be postponed, so I rallied to make the necessary provisions. A wonderful caregiver surfaced who my mom loved at first sight, for whom I gave my deep thanks to the universe, once again.

Once Mom's situation settled down, I made some time for me. I wanted to celebrate.

First, I wanted to see J again. Because of my fatigue, we had not been together since my treatment started. My reduced energy level concerned me a little, but I knew he'd understand if I wasn't as peppy as usual. I won't go into details, though I will say I thoroughly enjoyed returning to his arms. I brought him all sorts of information about radiation treatments, as I knew his scientifically curious mind would find that interesting. More importantly, I needed to talk about it and share with him.

After some time, we just laid back and enjoyed being close. As J continued to caress me, I watched his hand move over my body. Suddenly, I realized I felt nothing on my right breast, even though I could see him touching me there. Tears sprung to my eyes when I told him I was numb. I wanted so much to be back to "normal."

We tested the area again, and still nothing. He held me gently, assuring me that feeling would return. I thought he was merely appeasing me to be kind—but in fact, he was right. After all, the skin on the right side was still much darker than on the left, so more healing needed to happen.

I wish that other women suffering with the emotional aspects of breast cancer could have a lover as gentle and flirtatious as mine. I wish I could shout this out to the men in their lives, so the men would know how important is the comfort of their arms and their words of support. Through it all, J continued to remind me that he found me attractive and desirable—no matter what happened to my breast. I needed that very, very much.

Even though I was very disturbed by the after-effects of radiation, I never forgot that at least I still had my breast, and more importantly, I was alive and healthy! Eventually sensation returned, just as J said it would.

Traveling

By the time I went away over Memorial Day, everything was almost back to normal. I planned a multi-stop trip to visit several people I hadn't seen in some time. First, I went to Seattle to visit long-time friends. I had never been there, and had been promising to visit. I hadn't seen those folks for maybe 15 years or more. Mike (my date from my way-back high school prom) had just recuperated from prostate cancer. When we saw each other at a gathering for dinner, we just hugged and hugged, each of us with tears in our eyes. The best moment occurred when everyone else agreed that Mike and I, the two cancer survivors, looked the best of all. The gift of recovered health gave us survivors a special glow!

My friend Hannah's husband, Tom, had recently retired and proved an excellent guide to the wonders of his city during the day, while Hannah had to work. I had not really known him all that well before then. Hannah and I went to the same college, then worked together and became close friends while she lived in Chicago. She married Tom after moving to Seattle. I found it interesting that being open about something as intimate as my breast made it easier to feel closer to Tom. He took me on wonderful sight-seeing excursions to see the annual ritual of salmon swimming upstream, the beauty of the Japanese gardens, and the fun and variety of the market place. He was even patient while I shopped!

A friend of Tom's came to meet me, herself another survivor. She asked if my large muscle groups ached during radiation. Had she not asked, I never would have known what caused that pain. Instead, I would have continued to believe that radiation accelerated my aging process. That was another example of the importance of talking with others who share what you've gone through. So much to be learned, so much that the doctors themselves don't always know. As my oncologist said so frankly to me when I was diagnosed again the following year and questioning, seeking reasons: "…Betty, we know a lot more than we used to, but we don't know nearly enough about breast cancer." That goes for the effects of treatment, too. Of course, we are each unique beings. No one can know exactly how each individual will be affected.

My cousin Vicki met me in Seattle. From there, we drove on to a ferry—I've always wanted to be on one of those that take cars—to Victoria BC, where I found one of the loveliest, most romantic cities I've ever seen. Victoria is abundant with flowers, has a picturesque harbor and really friendly people. The Canadian dollar was weak compared to the American dollar, so everything seemed to be on sale—an added bonus for us. We stayed in a delightful bed and breakfast, where the couple who owned it brought us breakfast each morning. It was perfect to go to such a pretty place to celebrate my return to health, get waited on in luxury, and not even spend much money!

We returned via Port Angelis, Washington, and enjoyed short stops in Port Townsend and Portland, Oregon, before the long drive to Vicki's home in Eugene. After a couple of days there, I flew, happily, back home. A grand celebratory trip it was—and just part one of the celebrations I gave myself.

Six weeks later, I was off again. This time a long weekend in Eugene in early July, to attend the annual Oregon Country Fair—something I'd been promising myself for years. After coming through cancer, I felt that I now wanted to do everything I had always wanted to do, while I could.

An amazing, one-weekend-a-year event, the Country Fair is a throwback to the 60s, only drugs and alcohol are no longer allowed. A free bus ride from Eugene is when the experience begins, with most folks already talking and joking while standing in line. People of all kinds and all ages attend, many in various versions of costumes, or lack thereof—a man on stilts, a guy painted in silver, tattooed people, swimsuits over flesh-colored tights (for the synchronized swimmer parade), bare-breasted ladies with decorated bodies and big hats and feathers on their heads, a man wearing nothing but a couple of fanny packs (to cover his strategic parts) and a hat, kids in country fair costumes. There are events with jugglers, magicians, musicians, and speakers, as well as vendors at booths selling clothes and crafts and ice cream and foodstuffs and with environmental information and even a yurt! Music is everywhere. People are laughing and staring and dancing and walking and eating. It is totally and completely wacky fun.

I caught the spirit of the event right away, and if I had not just gone through surgery and radiation on my right breast, I might have ripped off my own shirt! That's how free it feels to be at this fair. Perfect celebration number two.

I returned home in time for my birthday the following week. My former mother-in-law came from California to visit. We are all that is left of her family, and she wanted to be reassured of my health. My granddaughter, Angie, and I usually celebrate our birthdays together, since they're one day apart. This year, celebration number three, we went to a spiffy French restaurant (after all, my birthday *is* on Bastille Day) where we had a great meal as well as special entertainment from a mime who took a shine to Angie. Few things make a grandma happier than watching her grandchild's face smiling in delight.

We culminated the evening with a special treat for Angie, who longed for a ride in a horse-drawn carriage. To Angie's delight, we climbed aboard for a ride around the city. How special for me to make a dream of hers come true.

My son still lived with me then, so we had a big pajama party with Grandma Vera in one bedroom, me in another, and Adam and Angie on the living room floor. What a fun time. We laughed and celebrated in a grand way; Adam was especially happy to see me healthy and energetic enough to travel and play again. I was pretty glad about it myself!

The end of March through July seemed an on-going celebration for me.

But life is a continuous cycle of up and down, yin and yang. The downturn happened when my friend Kathleen, who suffered so much with her own cancerous condition, left us late in August. Kathleen's spirit hung in there for me thanks to her collection of inspirational quotations which helped me so much during my second trial of breast cancer.

14

The First Fall

"Difficulties are meant to rouse, not discourage."

—William Ellery Channing

My energy returned gradually, and completely, and I jumped right back into my busy life.

Bit by bit my burnt, darkened skin sloughed off to give way to the emerging pink skin. The surgery had taken a golf-ball sized hunk out of my breast, so in addition to a scar, I had an indentation. Doctor Bill affectionately called it my "divot." Why did I think I heard a nurse tell me that it would fill in, eventually? Did I just imagine that because it's what I wanted to hear? Scar tissue also caused a hard spot which softened a bit over time, but still exists.

The shape, size and feel of my right breast were quite different than my left. I didn't really mind having a smaller, firmer breast—but I really DID mind that they were of such different sizes. I told myself that I was blessed to have kept both breasts, and that I shouldn't complain. Even though I felt guilty about such vanity, it really bothered me.

Life went on.

When I thought back on the experience, I believed there was something I was supposed to learn from it. Certainly, I had become more spiritual and more grateful for all the good things in my life compared with how I felt prior to having cancer. In addition, I had become more interested in and aware of good health and nutrition. Also, my perspective had changed, and I wanted to reach out more to help others.

But mostly, I went about the business of my life. As proud as I was of getting myself through the entire ordeal, simultaneously I just wanted to be done with it and put it behind me.

I jumped right back into packing my schedule, as usual, with teaching, client work, and family activities. My mom reached her 85th birthday that summer, and even though she needed a caregiver 24/7, she was able to enjoy the large party I gave for her with friends and family galore. We both had a lot to celebrate!

Right around that time, my son met Lisa, who became his wife. I saw less and less of him for a few weeks and then, suddenly, he called to tell me they'd be married in a matter of days! A whirlwind romance. More importantly, a great love for each of them. Adam married into a wonderful family who accepted him with open arms.

Both he and Lisa had daughters from their first marriages, and fortunately, the girls got along just fine and became close and loving sisters. As I write this, Adam and Lisa have just produced a baby boy—so it's a "yours, mine and ours" blended family.

What surprised me was how much I missed Adam. I liked having him around. I relied on the comfort of his company while I went through surgery and recuperation, and radiation and recuperation. And then, poof, he left. I had my second bedroom back as my full-time office, but I felt lonely. I realized I was experiencing the "empty nester" syndrome. Very weird for someone like me who treasures her privacy!

One of the things that changed in my life was admitting having needs that I couldn't always fulfill myself. I needed the love of my family and friends and at long last, allowed myself to rely on them to give that to me. I allowed myself to receive. Frankly, it felt very good to be open to what I used to consider weakness. Good to admit that although many think I'm a strong woman, I need those folks and their love...that caring in my life. It has always been difficult for me to even say "I need" and admit that I had a weakness—but I found that to be part of my humanity. Amazingly, once I actually said the words and asked for what I wanted and needed, I found I had a better chance of receiving it.

My doctor schedule consisted of quarterly visits, alternating between Dr. DJ, the breast surgeon, and Dr. Kathy, the oncologist. After two years, the appointments would take place semi-annually for three more years—a total of five years in all, taking Tamoxifen all the time. This drug is supposed to help prevent further breast cancers. There are potential side affects, of course, such as hot flashes, bleeding, vaginal discharge, and possible weight gain.

Once again, fortune smiled on me. I had few negative side effects from ceasing hormone replacement therapy (HRT) and from taking Tamoxifen, except for an increase in "flushes" (not too bad) and a tendency to hang onto unwanted weight.

My next annual mammogram was scheduled for December 14, almost a year after surgery. The exact anniversary would have been December 30, but we pushed it up to enable me to take a trip to Mexico over Christmas—another place I had never been. After years of struggling financially and therefore being unable to travel much, I finally had the wherewithal to fulfill some of my wander-lust and travel about the country and on occasion, abroad. Once each year I tried to go somewhere I had never been. The Mexico trip fulfilled my quest for a new place. It seemed a good way to end the year.

I felt some apprehension going for the mammogram, but told myself that was silly, just some deja vu feelings. After all, how could lightning strike twice? I was taking medication to protect me from further breast cancer. In fact, I didn't even think to ask anyone to come with me. What could happen?

To my horror, the technician returned to the examining room and said those dreaded words, "The doctor wants to see you in her office."

I walked into that office with dread. When the doctor appeared, I said, "This isn't going to be good, is it?" She solemnly replied, "It never is when you have to come in here."

In spite of the fact that I was on Tamoxifen, in spite of the fact that nothing showed up just one year prior—there it was, again, this time on the left side. The white, fuzzy spots on my film were very, very tiny, but they were there, definitely there.

Another biopsy had to be scheduled.

I couldn't decide if this should be before or after my holiday trip to Mexico. If it happened before and the results were positive, my trip would be ruined. Or, if I didn't even get the results before I left, I'd worry, and that could ruin my trip. On the other hand, I didn't want to have the procedure hanging over my head. Frankly, I just didn't want to face it, period.

I really did not want to believe this could happen again. But then, I didn't believe it could happen to me the first time, so why wouldn't it happen a second time?

Of course, I contacted J immediately. By this time, we were drifting apart. I wanted more from the relationship than he could give, and he had issues to deal with that had nothing to do with me. Still, we had a long and intimate history, and I needed his usually wise counsel. He advised me to go and have a good time, and deal with the biopsy on my return. I returned from Mexico on Dec. 28 and had the biopsy the next morning, Dec. 29.

It wasn't a very good December for me. The trip was not one I'd want to repeat. I didn't like the long Mexican bus ride that took us to a place I didn't enjoy very much, where they served food I didn't particularly care for (except for the guacamole, of course), and where the climate didn't agree with me (hot days/cold nights). Knowing I'd go back home to an unwanted procedure didn't help one bit, either.

I went to have the biopsy with a heavy heart. I felt doom hanging over my head, I missed J, my mother was declining, and I had no one waiting for me at home. Once again I had to wait over a long holiday weekend for results. Dr. DJ phoned me at 10:30 a.m. on January 3 to say, "positive." We scheduled an appointment for 7:30 a.m. on the first Friday of the New Year.

I called Sarah right away. I could barely talk as my throat filled with emotion, but I knew she, above all, would help me through this—again.

15

Same Song, Second Verse...

"Expecting the world to treat you fairly because you are a good person is a little like expecting the bull not to attack you because you are a vegetarian."

—*Dennis Wholey*

Sarah offered to accompany me for the appointment I didn't want to attend. I quickly accepted. Sarah knew that anxiety could cause me to block whatever the doctor told me, so she would act as my "recorder of information" and, of course, to bolster me. When she asked what else I'd like her to do, I told her that I wanted to see her face when I came out of surgery. Of course, she wouldn't have had it any other way. One thing I learned well was that I did not have to go through all this alone—a lesson for which I became increasingly grateful.

Having Sarah with me made all the difference. We had been through so much together, I found her presence comforting. I didn't want to think about going through all that again without her there every day, though I was glad she didn't have to endure it, herself. She suffered so much already in her own battles with breast and colon cancer.

Sarah was the only person to whom I voiced my secret concern. I asked her if she thought cancer struck again because God was punishing me for complaining that my right breast had become so much smaller than my left. Sarah set me straight at once, replying almost tersely, "My dear Betty, God isn't that petty!"

As coincidence would have it, Sarah and I were both patients of the same surgeon, Dr. DJ. She had a special relationship with him since he operated on her four times in one year for breast and colon cancer, and consequently, she felt no compunction about coming right in to the examining room with me.

Our doctor is a very busy man and has patients stacked up in the waiting room, as if in a holding pattern. The room isn't very large, and certainly doesn't seem big enough to hold the people who start streaming in. It seems just before they hit capacity, names start getting called.

Once a name is called, the patient goes into a small examining room where a nurse takes some information and then, more waiting. The doctor visits examining room after examining room, sometimes with a student in tow. I'm sure he expects to see each patient quietly sitting on the examining table, looking up expectantly when the doctor enters the room. Imagine his surprise when he saw both Sarah *and* me in the same room! He did a double take. At first, poor Dr. DJ didn't seem quite sure which of us to examine that day!

Of course, during the prior year's visits with him, both Sarah and I had told him about the sweet friendship we had developed during our period of radiation therapy. I think his eyes moistened when I first mentioned it. I know he was delighted to see two of his patients supporting each other so much.

Sarah paid close attention to everything the doctor said. Once again he was impressed with the mammographer's reading and called it a "good catch." Once again saying "DCIS" (ductal carcinoma in situ), tubular, sub-type, slightly invasive. I simply never understood how my cancer could be "in situ," in place, and at the same time be slightly invasive. But so it seemed. He also mentioned the possibility of taking lymph nodes, which did not happen the first time around.

The doctor explained to me that my left side constituted a second primary occurrence, not a recurrence. That was good news, in a way, translating to the fact that my original cancer hadn't spread. This second cancer was independent. This was a whole new tumor.

He set the date of surgery for January 18. Quickly, I thought. The last time I had more than a month's notice before surgery. This time I had less than two weeks—precious little time between the doctor visit and the operation. That worried me a little. Lots of things worried me.

Of course, I wondered about the effectiveness of Tamoxifen. But the fact is that the left-side tumor may have been there before I started the medication, just too tiny to show up on the film. In both cases, my incidents of cancer were microscopic, not at all palpable, and discovered early. I benefited from being faithful about my annual mammograms. In spite of the more recent controversy, I urge my female friends to get themselves checked regularly. I will never know if that actually saved my life, but I do know those yearly mammograms were responsible for the earliest detection.

Nurse Carole met with me separately and explained all that could happen, and what I would need to do for my post-op personal care if lymph nodes had to be removed. The possibility of waking up from surgery with a drain on my left side scared me. It drove me nuts that I couldn't know ahead of time whether or not this would happen. I don't know why of all things the drain thing bothered me so much, but it did.

The pre-op procedure changed since the year before. This time she told me I would have a wire inserted as before, but instead of immediately preceding surgery, that would be done the day before surgery. I'd have to go home with that wire sticking into my breast and try to sleep with it in place. In the morning I would first have the wire positioning checked before experiencing a new procedure wherein nuclear medicine would be injected into my left side to trace the lymph nodes. If they proved to be cancerous, the path to the malignancies would show clearly. I didn't like anything I heard during that meeting, except for the assurance that once again, I had an excellent prognosis.

All the changes from my prior year's experience made me nervous, since it wouldn't be exactly the same this time. Going into the unknown can be scary. Especially when people are going to be doing things to my body while I'm under anesthetic and completely out of it!

The nurse and I met in a room housing a special library of breast cancer books and videos—so I borrowed a video on yoga and took some information about Gilda's Club. This time, I was better informed than last time and thought it would be wise to prepare myself for the journey ahead. Additionally, I had become much more interested in overall health, inside and out, so I tried to learn more about nutrition and meditation.

This second time of cancer, I knew to raise my consciousness about what I had to learn. I believed that God was telling me something, maybe, "Okay, Betty, since you didn't get it the first time, I'm hitting you over the head with a hammer so you'll pay more attention."

Spreading the News

I was enormously touched by the effect my second round of cancer had on my friends and family. I welcomed the love and support that came from them.

Suzy burst into tears when she heard the news. Pat, who went through her own round the year before, told me how emotional she became when she next met with her oncologist, after hearing about my situation. True, she felt concern about me, but admitted feeling guilty being glad this hadn't happened to her. When she shared that with me, I told her I totally understood, and that I would have felt exactly the same way, though I didn't know if I'd have had the guts to admit it, as she did.

My dear son, Adam, did not take my announcement well. He and I love each other hugely and have seen each other through many of life's melodramas. I'm sure he started to worry about losing me. Even though he now lived with his wife some distance away, shortly after hearing that I had cancer again, he came for an ad hoc visit and just sort of hung around. I think he needed the comfort of seeing that I functioned normally, that outwardly I was looking and acting healthy. He needed to allay his fears. It felt good to have him near me.

One girlfriend immediately asked what she could do, two others who lived out of town offered to stay with me, and Pat immediately messengered me the "Breast Book" by Dr. Susan Love, which she had bought the year before but had never sent to me. This time I really needed it. I wanted to know everything I could about what was happening to me.

The e-mails came, the cards came, and the flowers came. Each day it cheered me to see them and to smell the flowers. There's something about fresh flowers that lift my spirits like nothing else. They are sunshine.

Because there were so many friends and family extra-concerned about my having a second bout with cancer, I wrote on-going e-mails to a group of close women friends which I entitled my "Boob Report." It helped me to communicate in that way—keeping my girlfriends in the information loop, while stemming a flow of phone calls I really did not want. These dear ladies gave me an outpouring of love and support, which I deeply appreciated, but I simply could not talk to each one and describe the same story over and over again. E-mail proved a godsend.

Barb, my neighbor and good friend, left the silliest stuffed cow animal in front of my door—to keep me company as I drove to my daily radiation treatments, again. I strapped that silly little bovine to the back seat of my car so I could see her in my rear-view mirror each day I drove to the hospital, chuckling at the sight.

Amy started an on-going postcard campaign to me with RX messages like: "RX funny movie"; "RX good books"; "RX nature"; "RX dance" and other tips for cheering up.

Keeping a Journal

Sarah told me I shouldn't approach this second occurrence as just a "bump in the road," corroborating that there was something I must learn from it. I began to keep a special journal. Much of what I'm writing here has been taken from that oh-so-important book.

I thought it might be enlightening to document my experiences, my feelings, and my inspirations. Since I'm a tactile person, the book had to both look and feel nice. My friend Suzy picked out exactly the right one; spiral bound so it would lay flat, which made it easy to write in, it had a soft/hard, velvety-feeling pressed cork cover.

I knew I'd need something handy to lift my spirits at odd times. I decided to keep in my journal all the positive messages, e-mails and cards with all their good thoughts and prayers. Should I happen to wake up in the middle of the night, feeling alone and scared or sad, I would only need to look in that book. That journal became my companion during the next three months. It really helped.

Later, through spiritual guidance, I came to believe that my mission in life is to share insights from my own experiences in order to help others. Maybe that's "it"—the thing I'm supposed to learn. I'll never know for sure, of course, but it feels right. I pray that documenting two years of my life during my own battle with cancer might help some other person get through it a little easier.

"Keep a gratitude diary: it will change your life."

—Oprah Winfrey

16

Pre-Op Number Two

"Don't ever become a pessimist, Ira; a pessimist is correct oftener than an optimist, but an optimist has more fun—and neither can stop the march of events."

—Robert A. Heinlein, Time Enough for Love

Other than cancer, I was in great condition!

I went to my internist for all the pre-op tests, and surprisingly, my blood pressure was 110/78. Go figure. Had I really learned to put my mind in a quiet place, put my trust in the universe, in spite of the fact that I had cancer surgery looming over me again?

I threw myself into work from the beginning of January until right before surgery on January 18. Intense work that required serious concentration was a palliative against my fears.

At home on weekends, I busied myself with chores—straightened up my office, did laundry and went to movies. In fact, I went to a movie almost every day for each of the 5 days preceding surgery. Movies took me out of my own life. The big screen captivated me and became my whole world. For two or three hours each day, I was somewhere else. Cinema therapy.

For my last "free" evening, I visited with dear friends for some laughs, some wine and for the piece de resistance, holding their infant son. Nothing feels sweeter than an armful of loving child. When I heard that I might need to have a drain on my left side, I thought, "How will I hold the baby?" I thought of how I'd miss being able to pick him up and cuddle him. I was driving my car at the time and had to pull over when the tears came.

I enjoyed my movie-therapy alone, as I did not want to socialize with anyone. On the other hand, I wanted very much to be hugged. Adam wasn't there to give me one, and J was in another state (both physically and emotionally). I got weepy driving to my client, feeling sorry for myself. Fortunately, the woman I worked with, Meg, a good friend and survivor herself—and one of the people who inspired me to write all this—seemed to intuit what I needed. She greeted me with a huge hug that morning, and oh boy, did I ever need it.

As surgery loomed closer, I extracted myself from being totally enmeshed in work so I'd have a clearer schedule afterward. I wanted to pave the way for self-indulgence.

Friends called to try to cheer me. Adrienne, my best friend from high school and a transplant survivor, gave me encouragement when she phoned from Florida while visiting family. While she was gone, her husband insisted on taking me out to dinner and theater to keep me from hiding under my pillow. He happened to phone on the very night I received my diagnosis. When he innocently asked how I was, I responded by telling him I had cancer again and that I had been in bed with the covers over my head where I fully intended to stay until I absolutely had to come out. He said, "No, you're not going to do that. I love you, my wife loves you. You will get through this and for starters, we're going out for dinner. Tonight. So get dressed and be ready by 7." I gave in and was glad I did. It was much better going out and talking about books and life and even arguing than staying in bed, hiding.

My neighbor, Barb, called to let me know she would be home and available to me the night after my surgery. I told myself I didn't really want a babysitter. Truthfully, however, it was comforting to know she'd be around. Bit by bit I let people do more for me. I was learning to accept the goodness of others.

I became increasingly grateful for my friends and their love and support. We don't always get to know how others feel about us, not really. My friends were telling me, in their various ways, of their love. How blessed I felt.

I allowed the tears to flow. They often came at unexpected times—driving my car, or in the shower. One day while bathing, I held my left breast and looked at the bruise from the biopsy, knowing there was more to come for that poor boob, and I cried and cried. Betty Rollins was only partly right with "First you cry." I thought, "Yes, and then you cry some more and some more and some more."

I kept thinking about the surgery, dreading the pain and discomfort I knew would come and most of all, dreading the disruption to my life! I thought of not only the recuperation from the surgery itself, but also all that would follow. I thought of returning to radiation therapy, going there every single day again, and then the suffering from exhaustion, burned skin and foggy brain.

Sandy, the friend who went with me for my first biopsy the prior year, took me to the wire insertion procedure the afternoon before surgery. Since she had been a nurse, I knew she wouldn't get queasy, though I thought I might. I expected it to be horrible going home from the medical center with a piece of metal sticking out of my breast. I was wrong. They taped the wire securely, so that it neither protruded nor caused discomfort. Since there turned out to be no reason to go right back home and hide my top half, Sandy and I figured, "What the heck?" We took ourselves to a movie (the fifth day in a row for me). Afterward, we bumped into some women I knew. Since I had till midnight before I needed to stop food and liquids, we all went to dinner. This unexpected evening took my mind off the next day and became a spontaneous celebration of life at the moment—in the long run, what we have at the moment is all we really can count on.

17

Reprise—Surgery Number Two

○ ○

"Never grow a wishbone, daughter, where your backbone ought to be."

—Clementine Paddleford

I woke up early in the morning, pleasantly surprised to see that the wire remained in my left breast and hadn't seemed to move one iota during the night. I don't know why I had no trouble zonking out the night before—I thought sleep would have been difficult, but not so. I think I was able to put my mind somewhere else for the time being, which kept me from anxiety. Or maybe I just like to sleep! I thoroughly enjoyed my shower. Even though I had to be careful of the wire and the adhesive holding it in place, I knew from my last experience that it could be awhile before I'd be able to really enjoy a shower again.

The schedule for the day ahead did not please me. Although my surgery wasn't scheduled until noon, I had to be at the hospital by 7:45 a.m. for pre-op procedures—first, the wire-check, then nuclear medicine by 8:00 a.m. That meant I'd have a half day to wait and wait, without even a cup of coffee. I am not a patient person—I just hate waiting. There was nothing I could do about it, so I resigned myself to the schedule and made sure to bring a good book in order to pass the time enjoyably.

Suzy picked me up about 7:00 a.m. to take me to the hospital. I'm reminded, now, of how many friends I mention within these pages. I did not want to burden anyone with my problems, but so many offered to help. Especially this time, the second time around. So I sort of spread it about, amongst several people. That way, I wouldn't be asking too much of any individual. Still, I wondered how I would ever pay them all back for their kindnesses? I told myself that life is cyclical and that paying back might not be a direct route. Perhaps I'd be able to help others as my life goes on. Paying it forward, as they say.

First, we made a quick stop at the mammography center to ensure the wire remained exactly where it needed to be. It did. This was important since that wire would guide the surgeon to the very spot of my tumor. The last time, the cancer sat deep inside, almost at the wall of my chest. This time, the spot was closer to the front of my breast, so I definitely would not have matching incisions—though I didn't let myself worry about that. All I could think of was whether or not I'd wake up with that drain in my armpit.

I moved on to my 8:00 a.m. appointment in nuclear medicine. The nuclear medicine offices share the same waiting room with the radiation offices. That's where Sarah and I agreed to meet, once again. Emotions started to well up in me as Suzy and I walked into that waiting room, after having been there every single weekday for six-and-a-half weeks barely a year before. Seeing Sarah, with her sunshine-bright smile and arms opening wide, I felt infinitely better. Becky, a radiation technician who had been part of our team, came in to escort a patient into the rooms and did a double-take when she saw the two of us standing there. Her face lit up, as we really had brought some joy to those rooms, but her expression quickly changed when she noticed that I wore a hospital gown.

I felt reassured knowing that Becky would be there for me again. Most of the team that we knew had already moved on. There must be a high burn-out rate for the wonderful kids on the radiation tech teams. They see so much mutilation from cancer surgeries every single day, yet they always approach each patient cheerfully and professionally, making each of us feel welcome and special.

I was soon called in to have a radioactive dye injected that would highlight my lymph nodes. The nuclear medicine rooms were foreboding, of course. Even though I thought I knew my way around that part of the hospital, I had never been in this particular area. All the medical professionals were scurrying about in their workday surroundings. New patients like me found it unfamiliar, overwhelming, and sterile.

Another new thing, another mystery, another huge machine that dwarfed me. I thought of the little, tiny human found in Japanese landscapes that illustrate man's insignificance in relation to the universe.

The radioactive dye was a new procedure to me. Because of on-going breast cancer studies, the "standard operating procedure" changes year after year as more is learned about breast cancer. The dye would not only show the exact location of the nodes, but it would also highlight the difference between the benign and, God forbid, the malignant ones, if any. Mostly, I just held my breath, gritted my teeth, and told myself that this moment would soon pass, that nothing lasts forever, and I willed myself to be brave. Actually, it really wasn't bad at all, just different and more of the unknown. I watched the whole process on a big monitor. I couldn't really figure out what the doctor explained, though I tried to appear as intelligent as I could. I wonder why it seemed important to me to try to impress him with my good brain, as if being a "good girl" somehow would ensure better results. For some inane reason I really tried to get that doctor to like me, as if whether or not he liked me would affect the outcome. It reminded me of playing the student-teacher game to get a good grade.

How much of our lives have been affected by our approach to grades in the school system, I wonder? There I was, lying flat on my back, receiving nuclear medicine from a doctor I'd never see again, trying to make him like me so he'd give me a good grade!

It ended rather painlessly after all. I was just putting the gown back on to cover the top half of my body (they let me keep my pants on for the procedure) when all of a sudden a nurse appeared, handed me a different hospital gown, and said "Undress completely and get this clean gown on, the gurney's on the way." I was blessed! Surgery had been pushed up and they were ready for me right that minute. So much for my earlier concerns about waiting for hours—and another lesson in acceptance for me. Now that my consciousness has been raised, I realize that the more I allow myself to accept and the less I try to control, the easier life becomes. Maybe I should repeat the serenity prayer to myself multiple times each day!

Things started happening quickly. The gurney arrived almost the minute I donned the clean gown. Someone got Suzy and Sarah from the waiting room so they could bring my personal belongings and accompany me to the surgery floor. They barely squeezed on to the same elevator with me on the gurney and my attendant. As soon as the elevator doors opened, they were told to go one way, while my attendant wheeled me in the opposite direction.

Things were happening fast in pre-op.

The anesthesiologist appeared immediately to quiz me. The rest of the team began gathering around, repeating many of the same questions over and over. Somebody said, "Where's your wrist bracelet?" and then yelled, "She doesn't have her wrist bracelet!," as if it were my fault that no one put one on me. This felt like a crash team, which was a bit unnerving. The wrist bracelet appeared, as did my breast surgeon. Things started to calm down. It seemed as if everything was suddenly under control the minute Dr. DJ arrived. He smiled down at me, his blue eyes full of kindness and compassion and, I thought, filled with confidence. It gave ME confidence. I put my trust in him once again. After all, we were getting to be old friends.

I remember being wheeled into a chilly operating room and shifting from the gurney to a narrow operating table. People were connecting monitoring devices to me and IVs. I noticed a bright light and a bunch of faces before passing out.

I woke up in a bed in a real hospital room this time, not just a recovery room as before. A nurse leaned over me, making sure I was warm enough. The combination of the coolness in the operating room (I've been told they keep it that way so the doctors don't perspire too much) and the shock to my system gave me horrible shakes after surgery. I needed lots of extra blankets. I thought back to another time years ago when I came out of an outpatient surgery and my mom was hovering over me in the recovery room, worrying about my uncontrollable trembling. She piled blankets on top of me and then laid as much of her own body as she could on top of that, in order to generate more heat. Even though I told her not to come to the hospital this time since she could barely walk anymore, deep down I wanted her there.

As soon as I could speak, I asked the attending nurse if I had a drain. Much to my surprise, she didn't even know. Of course, I thought this would be the most important thing to everyone! But then, how would anyone else know my own personal dread fear? She lifted the covers as I winced and braced myself and said, "No, nothing. No drain." Tears flowed from relief.

Suzy and Sarah came in smiling warmly, anxious about how I felt, and looking relieved. The doctor told them all went well. In addition to excising the tumor, he removed only two sentinel nodes from under my arm and both were benign. Phew!

Since all was well, we insisted that Suzy keep her lunch date. Sarah stayed with me. With her help, I got dressed to go home. I was still a little woozy, so I sat on the edge of the bed for a bit. Sarah bent toward me, unpinned her angel and put it on my jacket. She said, "I told you this is for you. She'll watch over you now and for as long as you need." That little angel stayed with me for some time to come until I believed some one else needed her more than I did.

I have kept my belief in angels. They are always with me now, always supporting me, always there when I need them.

We left the hospital even though my body felt a little wobbly, and my throat was killing me from the tube that had been inserted during the anesthetic. It was wonderful to get back to the familiarity of my own home, the place I love to be more than anywhere else.

Sarah stayed with me. Even though I went directly to bed, her nearby presence comforted me. I told her she could leave, of course, but she refused to do that until the next care-person arrived. Barb, my neighbor-friend, left work early that day to be with me and appeared at my door late that afternoon with an entire shopping cart full of foodstuffs she brought to make meals for me.

Once Sarah met Barb and felt assured that I would be in good hands, she agreed to go home. I got out of bed to say goodbye and thanks, and decided to sit in the kitchen while Barb made me a healthy, easy to swallow dinner—poached salmon, steamed vegetables and fresh bakery bread—before giving me a pain killer and pushing me back to bed. She offered to spend the night, but I told her since she lived so close, I'd phone if I needed help. She busied herself in my kitchen, cooking vegetable soup for the next day. From time to time, I'd be aware of kitchen sounds through my drugged stupor. Occasionally my eyes opened, and I'd see a light from the front room. I have no idea how late Barb stayed that night. I know I felt totally cared for and secure with someone watching over me like that.

The next day, Friday, my favorite aunt, Cookie, arrived purportedly to make me lunch and care for me. The truth is, we both just napped! Our family has strong sleep genes. We all love to sleep and we love our naps. Cookie took the couch and I stayed in bed. It was wonderful to have her near, though there was precious little to do other than sleep or sit and eat.

Comfort like that only comes from the dear ones in our lives. My aunt is as close to a sister as I'll ever have, since I'm an only child. My mom had four siblings born over a 20 year span—two siblings older than mom, and two siblings younger than mom. Cookie, mom's baby sister, was 13 years younger than mom and 13 years older than me. (And I was 13 years older than Cookie's daughter. The four of us liked that connection.)

Cookie was not a healthy person, so her husband had to drive her everywhere. I'm sure he didn't mind the long drive from their suburban home to my home in the city to bring Cookie to me the day after breast cancer surgery. My uncle was especially supportive, having undergone a male mastectomy himself a few years earlier. One thing about cancer, it creates quite a bond among us survivors.

My kids came by, also. Adam needed to see me to be sure I looked all right. His wife, Lisa, prepared lunch and waited on us, serving the soup that Barb cooked the night before. Nice, very nice.

My left underarm was very sore and hurt whenever I moved it. As much as I dislike taking drugs, I stayed on Vicodin to deaden the pain. Fortunately, a thoughtful survivor made little pillows that the doctor's office gave to us when we were about to have incisions under our arms. I kept that soft pillow between my arm and side so that my arm didn't come down hard, aggravating the sore spot.

My mother stopped by with her caregiver. Mom had difficulty walking, but I knew she needed to see me for herself—just like my son. She did a good job juggling her concern for me with knowing I didn't like being "fussed" over. She was wonderful at appearing to be energetic and optimistic—traits she held on to until the last several weeks of her life. She had one of those "the show must go on" spirits, which she made contagious. Being a good Jewish mother, Mom brought chicken soup and sandwiches. I lasted about an hour with her, before I needed to get back to bed. The painkillers were knocking me out.

Amazingly, by Saturday morning—just two days after surgery—the pain had diminished so drastically that I could shower, very carefully of course, and even wash and blow dry my hair. I experimented with using my left arm to hold the hair dryer and to my delight, it worked just fine! I'm sure every woman knows how much better we feel when our hair looks good.

It took some courage to look at the surgery site, but all I saw were surgi-strips (adhesive strips), no bruising yet, and some slightly bloody strings under my arm. Not nearly as ghastly as I thought it would be.

I enjoyed a lovely Saturday home alone watching movies and reading. Just what the doctor ordered, so to speak. My mind was pretty much at ease, since I already knew the sentinel nodes were negative, though I still had to wait for the pathology report regarding the removed tumor and its surrounding area. I went to sleep early that night, already able to lie on my left side, quite relieved to be healing so quickly. I remained alone on Sunday, enjoying drinking coffee, reading the newspaper for hours, and resting.

18

Post-Op Number Two

By Monday, I felt much better, though still weak. During the long periods of quiet time over the weekend, my thoughts had gone inward. I felt that I had been "touched" by cancer—not just physically, but in a way that goes beyond that. It was something I didn't know or pay attention to before I had been afflicted.

I knew I needed to adopt a healthier lifestyle—to be more conscious about what I ate, to get regular exercise, to better balance all the aspects of my life, to reduce stress and to allow myself quiet time to just "be." Those were starters.

I learned more about meditating, continued with my journaling, and tried to learn to take time for myself without feeling guilty.

Late that afternoon, walking about my quiet home, I heard a weird sort of "sloshing" sound. I tried to stop and stand perfectly still in order to hear where it came from. I noticed that every time I stopped, it stopped. I deduced that the sound was coming from ME, more specifically, from my left breast!

To be sure, I tested it. I stood still, then stomped my foot. Slosh. I hopped (gently)—slosh. I sat down and got up quickly—slosh. What WAS that? Why was there liquid inside my breast? Should I have had the drain? Should I visit the doctor so he could suction it off? I didn't know what to do. I fretted all evening. First thing the next morning, I called the doctor's office and anxiously waited for a return call.

Nurse Beth phoned. She told me good news about my pathology report: the "margins were clear." Fortunately, this time I knew what that meant. I had a .4cm tumor, which was very, very tiny; the area around it showed no sign of additional cancer. A golf-ball sized area had been removed which explained the empty hole that was now inside my left breast. I know this may sound like a surgeon's over-reaction to a microscopic tumor, and maybe he was being overly careful. I assumed my doctor played it cautious as he didn't want to have to go in again, something that happened to several other ladies I met in the waiting room. First they had surgery one, then after the path report, they had a second surgery in the same place to clear the margins. Not fun! Once is enough—believe me.

That new hole in my breast, Beth explained, had filled up with liquid from my body—remember, nature abhors a vacuum. She said, eventually, the liquid would be absorbed and the sloshing would disappear. I didn't really believe her.

I was still feeling a little shaky that day, but I had been housebound since Friday afternoon—and enough is enough. My very special friend, Michael, asked to stay with me before he returned to Europe, where a new job waited for him in Paris. Michael is one of the dearest men in my life. He is as comfortable to be with as a brother, and attractive enough to enjoy flirting with him. We adore each other, though years back made the unspoken decision to keep our relationship on a friendship-only basis. He is not only handsome and humorous, but also a thoughtful man who makes me feel good as a person, a friend, and as a woman. What more could I ask for? Plus, he's one of those men who just loves boobs—on real women, on statues, in art, wherever. So he was particularly concerned about me and mine.

The fresh air helped me a great deal when I went to the airport to greet him. Plus, I needed the diversion from my concerns about "sloshing." It was wonderful to see Michael, though I had to ask him not to hug too tightly (he's a really good hugger, but this was not the time for the big kahuna).

I really enjoyed his company. Michael had plenty of personal things to attend to during the day since he had fairly recently moved from Chicago to Paris. That gave me clear days to myself and Michael's company each evening for dinner and conversation. Lovely. I still tired easily, so we didn't go out much. One night, though, we met a mutual friend at a new restaurant with whom we talked and laughed. Though it was a bit too soon for me to go out and socialize, I think I put up a good show and hung in there fairly well. We got back later than expected, feeling relaxed from the wine we drank. For a long time we sat in my darkened living room, holding hands and talking. I treasure that memory.

Those sloshing sounds made me self conscious. Fortunately, Michael and I have been close for years, and I could be candid with him. I asked him straight out if he could hear my breast "sloshing." He broke into laughter and said something like, "You know I love everything about those boobs of yours, whether they make noise or not! Relax, the sloshing will go away." He also told me he couldn't hear it at all, even though I made him lean his head towards my chest to listen. That made me feel better, whether or not it was true.

We had a wonderful time together that first week after my surgery, and it took my mind off any of those feeling-sorry-for-myself moments. On Michael's last night in the states, he cooked us a marvelous dinner. His own special stir-fry is a favorite of mine. And then he asked me on which day of the week my birthday would fall this year. I checked a calendar and told him it would be a Saturday. He said, "Then come to Paris!"

It didn't take me long to make those plane reservations. What a grand idea. One that turned out to be an absolutely, incredibly fantastic birthday!

I took Michael to O'Hare International airport one week after he arrived. By that time, I felt much more like my old self. Although I was excited for him and his new Parisian opportunity, I hated to see him leave.

When I returned home, I went back to my old ways of worry—would I be able to regenerate my work after taking off so long, what should I do about money, should I stop spending unnecessarily and going out to restaurants? Was it really not even two weeks since surgery?

One night in bed trying to get comfy, I attempted to bring my arm over my head and found I just couldn't do it. I worried that my arm would never work the same again. The skin felt tight, as if there wasn't quite enough to allow my arm to reach up. After that, I tried to remember to stretch my arms up high several times a day. I could actually feel the left side stiffening if I neglected that exercise.

Later, of course, I realized most of my concerns were unfounded. The regular stretching ensured the return of my range of motion, and my clients had just been letting me recover—they hadn't disappeared. The money came back when the work returned, I could go to out to eat without worrying about the expense, I continued exercising, and life went on.

Some concerns remained, of course. At my post-op doctor appointment, Dr. DJ told me all went well. However, when I asked him if I'd be prone to breast cancer the rest of my life, he just shrugged his shoulders. The fear of this being a chronic condition remains, albeit to a lesser degree each year. However, my mind and soul are at a different place now than before my first diagnosis and if the worst, physically, should happen, I know I will be able to find the necessary inner strength.

19

Gilda's Club

○ ○

"There are things that are so serious that you can only joke about them."

—Helsenberg

Again, I had about a month between surgery and the start of my second go-round with radiation. This time, I wanted to better prepare myself for what I knew was ahead.

The first thing I did was sign up at Gilda's Club. This amazing place is a cancer support community named for the famous comedienne, Gilda Radner, who died of ovarian cancer. There are sixteen Clubs across North America. I did not feel the need for this the first time I had cancer, thinking I'd get through it, be done with it, and go on with my life.

This time, I knew the effect on my life would be deep. Lightning had struck twice, which made me feel as if I had been clobbered in order to make me more aware. I wasn't sure what that meant, but I could no longer avoid connecting myself with being a cancer patient. I could not blow off the prior year anymore with a "Phew, that's over!" and merely go on with my life. This time I knew I had to pay attention. I believed Sarah when she told me this was more than a bump in the road for me.

I thought I'd want additional support and so I set out to establish a safety net before I actually had a NEED. To that end, I read that little brochure about Gilda's Club that I saw in the doctor's office and the radiation therapy waiting room. I called that particular support center because it was the most convenient location to my home. The experience with Gilda's Club was amazing. I actually felt privileged to become part of it. They make us cancer people feel so special, without ever being condescending or over-protective.

I recommend finding a support group to everyone whose life is affected by cancer. It's not just one of those "oh, you poor thing" situations, but instead, insightful guidance by experienced people who help you get through a life-altering experience. Most of us can get through it on our own, of course—but why not make it easier? There are no extra points for being a martyr!

I made an appointment on a Saturday morning for an orientation and personal interview. The Club in Chicago is located in a very popular area, squeezed in between a couple of "hot" restaurants, and completely unrecognizable except for its bright red door. Once they buzzed me in, I found myself in a pleasant reception area, replete with Gilda Radner posters, photos and quotes—all over the place. Everyone who works there—either paid or volunteer—is nice. Really, really nice.

I joined a small group of cancer people (fellow patients, survivors, family members). Together, we were welcomed and given the tour of the facilities—everything from kitchens (plural—they told us that food is a large issue with cancer patients because we either eat for comfort, or can't eat due to illness), children's play areas ("Noogieland"—Gilda called kids "noogies"), meeting areas and private rooms for talking or being quiet or reading. There were also larger group meeting rooms, including one named the "It's always something" room. Gilda used to say, "It's always something…if it's not one thing, it's another…" I was told support groups were available, as were family sessions, and that there were activities like yoga, art, specific types of cancer networking nights, healthy cooking classes and so on. I could even just flop there and read if I had some hours to kill between business meetings. I was invited to consider this "my" place.

There are no fees for membership in Gilda's Club, nor do they hit on members for donations. The thinking is that people affected by cancer already have enough to deal with without being asked for money. That philosophy touched me deeply. They understand how deeply we were affected by this rotten disease. They cared. They were there to help us.

I met privately with an intake counselor who created a customized membership plan for me. I told her I had become more interested in overall health and nutrition—healthier food, appropriate vitamins and supplements, and regular exercise. When I saw that Gilda's Club had a class on Dr. Andrew Weil's book, "Eight Weeks to Optimum Health," she signed me up immediately.

What an experience. The teacher, Tom, was a survivor himself. He had totally changed his life from the high-pressure environment he had before his illness to now being a healthy life coach, personal trainer, and teacher of this wonderful course. Each week, we cancer people of all ages, all races, all degrees of treatment, came together while Tom got us involved in helping him cook a fun, tasty, and nutritious meal. While we were eating, he'd talk about the food-of-the-week and then took us through stretching exercises, played special, relaxing music for us, and guided us, chapter by chapter, on how to optimize our health in every way. Tom led us from taking a break from the world (a news fast) to keeping fresh flowers in our homes, as well as to suggestions on exercise, which vitamins and supplements to take, what foods to incorporate into our diets, and which to avoid.

We often joked about our situations. Tom called this "tumor humor." No matter, we laughed. Laughter is one fine medication.

I knew I didn't have a full eight weeks before the onset of my radiation treatments, but I decided to do what I could in the time available. It became so important and helpful to me that although it was an hour's drive from the hospital, I went to those classes even after treatment began, no matter how tired I felt.

The experience I had at Gilda's Club, especially in that eight-week class, supported my efforts to lighten my work load as well as to become more spiritual. I raised my awareness of what I put into my mouth, continued to stretch, started daily meditation, and made sure to journal most mornings. To this day, I try to back off from the toxicity of stress.

Later, I realized that Gilda's Club was a bit like my experience living in Israel the year after I graduated college. In Israel, being Jewish was the norm. Wherever I went I felt like I belonged, as if the whole country was peopled by an extended family of sorts.

All my childhood I lived in a predominantly Jewish environment, so it wasn't until I went to college and got out into the world that I realized what it meant to be singled out as a minority. One boy's father refused to let him date me; a sorority's by-laws denied their accepting me; and the company I worked for had a limited number of Jews, so taking time off for our Holy Days resulted in negative visibility.

But in Israel, all things about my heritage were openly accepted, everywhere. I had similar feelings about acceptance at Gilda's Club—except the commonality is cancer.

I only go to Gilda's Club on occasion these days. When I do stop in for yoga or cooking class or a special event, the welcome remains. I know that the folks at Gilda's Club are there for me whenever I wish. It is a wonderful place for cancer people, welcoming them and theirs with open arms, optimism and comfort.

20

Radiation Redux

o o o o o o o o o o o o o o o o o o o o o o o o o o o o o o o o o o o o o

"If you do what you've always done, you'll get what you've always gotten."

—*Anon*

During my pre-treatment appointment with the radiation oncologist, the good Doctor Bill, I shared my concerns about the potential of chronic breast cancer. He happens to be one great guy who calls it like he sees it, a quality that I really appreciate. He said my body produced in my left breast what it produced in my right breast, and "We took care of one side, now we'll take care of the other side. Unless you're hiding a third breast on me, you should be just fine. Plus, after this round of radiation, they should be closer to the same size." Hah! Cosmetic radiation!

Dr. Bill asked about my life in general, and we discussed my radiation schedule. We set up a time for the "simulation," the measurements, which I now know is how the process begins.

I appreciated having full energy during the weeks before returning to radiation, and I wanted to cling to it, as if that were possible. I wanted to do everything, see everyone, get everything done, get totally organized, and on the way, work on becoming more physically fit. Tall order! Of course, I did just a part of each—but it felt good to try.

This time I learned from the last time. I allowed myself not to pretend to always be so brave. I learned to clear my schedule as much as possible. I learned to ask for and accept help from the many friends who offered it. I learned to plan ahead for positive things that would overcome some of the difficult times. I learned that I had to make special efforts to reduce stress in my life.

My simulation was scheduled for Friday morning, Feb. 23…barely five weeks after surgery. I approached it with trepidation, remembering the severe discomfort from last time, as well as the subsequent 33 daily radiation treatments and their consequences.

Important things in my life had changed. The more I see, the more I realize that's how life happens. Nothing stays the same—good or bad. Nothing lasts forever. This time I was more alone, physically. I no longer had my son around for morning hugs, and my romantic relationship was ebbing away. Also, my mother's aging process was rapidly accelerating. I wanted to spend more time with her; I also wanted to spend more time with my granddaughter, Angie—I had become used to seeing her weekly when her dad lived with me and I missed her.

The key people who had been there for me during Round One were no longer there in the same way during Round Two. My anxiety level was high, even interrupting my sleep. This was especially disturbing to me, and I resented being robbed of this pleasure.

I reduced my work load drastically. I knew what lay ahead, and I knew how long it would last. I knew that I'd be foolish to continue to overload myself with work during that period. The work could be put off. I had to take care of myself, first.

I allowed myself to rely more and more on the many friends who offered their help and support. It was there for the asking, so I asked.

Before the simulation began, I told the technician of the horrible discomfort I suffered the last time. She found a way to support my arm and made me more comfortable during the entire process.

I asked Sarah to meet me for lunch afterwards. I knew that just returning to that room would be difficult. Even so, I hadn't prepared myself for how deeply depressing it would be afterwards to see those black felt tip pen markings surrounding my breast. They were a vivid, ugly reminder that I was repeating everything I went through a year earlier. Very "here-we-go-again." Fortunately, I could share those feelings with Sarah, who understood completely.

I named my angel pin "Annie" for my late, beloved grandmother. Her name was Anna, and she gave me unconditional love from the day I was born. After I told Sarah about my choice of the angel's name, she told me that she had chosen "Patience" for her angel name. Perfect on both counts.

That weekend, I returned to my movie therapy, and then immersed myself in reading, enjoying the silence in my home.

I did not want to face the first radiation treatment alone, so I asked a friend, the lovely Juliet, to take me. I dreaded going there every day knowing I wouldn't see Sarah; knowing I would have an unfamiliar tech team; knowing it would be another six-and-a-half weeks of daily treatments; knowing I would be losing my energy soon, and knowing my skin would start showing the effects of the burn.

Juliet responded, "Thank you for asking. I love you, and I've been wanting to do something to help. I just didn't know what to do." I learned from this sweet and very special young woman that people want very much to help; we just need to tell them how. They really want us to let them in.

I started treatment on Feb. 27. Thank God I had those tattoos that clearly marked the radiated area from the first time to ensure that I had no overlapping zapping.

The first night after treatment I slept from 9:15 p.m. all the way through to 8:00 a.m. It couldn't be that I'd already be feeling the effects, but nothing is impossible psychologically, so maybe that's what happened. I wanted to know why I slept so much that night. I pondered whether I was bored with my reduced work load. Or escaping? Or was my body anticipating a future reaction? What was going on?

I've been told that we need sleep to sort of re-set our bodies, much like a computer does when it's turned off and then back on. I've also been told that sleep is when the angels commune with us, when they nurture and heal us. Who knows? All I know for sure is it did wonders for me that night.

By the weekend, my energy seemed to be normal. Perhaps what I experienced earlier in the week had been psychosomatic? Perhaps my mind was jumping the gun, knowing that fatigue and cloggy-brain were waiting just around the corner.

I needed some inspiration and, fortunately, came across the collection from my late friend Kathleen's memorial service which helped me in many ways. One of her quotes gave me permission to just "hang out." Until now, this had been an alien concept to me, but I decided to try it.

Rachel

My long-time friend, Rachel, came to visit. Usually when Rachel visits, we just hang around and often go out to eat. This time, she accompanied me to my radiation treatment, and then I took her with me to my class at Gilda's Club.

Rachel and I go back to our high school days, so we've been in each other's lives for a long, long time. She moved away many years back. Our lifestyles are very different. She is beautiful and very natural with thick, long hair of its own color. She wears no make-up, doesn't own a business suit, likes to live far from any major city and lives very simply. I, on the other hand, am more of a city girl. Still, we remained in contact, sometimes closely, sometimes not; at one point, there was even a lengthy hiatus. Now, we are closer than ever. Our history is a strong bond.

We have comforted each other through so much of the ups and downs of life—from the girly-stuff of being roommates, through life-style changes, romances and heartbreak, to births, child-raising, severe illness, deaths and divorces. We've learned how to open ourselves to each other. We gut talk, we're supportive, and we're there for each other whenever there is a need. Often we end up abandoning ourselves, erupting in outrageous laughter.

Rachel lives on a limited income and watches her expenses very, very carefully. I really appreciated the fact that she spent the money on airfare to come visit me. It meant a lot that she accompanied me to and from treatment and class at Gilda's Club, but mostly, that she just hung around with me for a few days.

Ebb and Flow

Good things and bad things continued to flow in and out of my life. My work-load had decreased drastically, not all of my own doing, and the decreased income concerned me. As a self-employed person, I had no regular paycheck coming in; I earned my money from billable hours. During this second go-round, I started thinking about reviewing my life to assess what I'd been doing and what I'd like to do. Maybe I should make some drastic changes and find another source of income, a different way of life? Out of the blue, one client called and asked me to be on retainer. Right after that, the university asked that I teach another class. My cash flow problems began to diminish. Soon, I realized that I really did like what I do and the way I did it. I just needed more work.

Sometimes the answer is right there in front of you all the time.

Meanwhile, in addition to my anxiety about the effects treatment would have on me, I had a great deal of concern about my lover. I sensed major conflicts on his end at the same time that my own energy level and psyche weren't doing very well.

There is no point in dwelling on this, as what later happened to us had more to do with him than with me—and this is my story. Suffice it to say that we came

apart. J was in the midst of a severe mid-life crisis. That life event is so very difficult, yet can be so incredibly important in forcing us to look at who we really are,
who we want to be, and hopefully, allowing us to choose how to live our lives
after a mid-life correction.

I found it therapeutic to socialize with really close girlfriends. Especially with
the raucous laughter there is with my group. There's just something about close
girlfriends that can't be beat. They understand. They support. They might cook
for you or shop for you or even do your laundry. They understand about flowers.
They let you cry. And they get you to laugh.

As treatment progressed, by each Friday I'd get a sinking spell. And I began to
hurt. This time there was pain under my arm where I now had a scar from the
sentinel node removal. I longed for each weekend, knowing I'd have two whole
days of peace from being zapped—hoping my poor skin would heal a bit over
that brief time before my Monday appointment. I started putting special care
cream on my breast immediately after radiation, even before I noticed anything
too pink. It helped a lot.

I continued to get encouraging e-mails, cards and phone messages. Meg told
me "A positive mental attitude is the elixir of life." I wrote that in my journal and
tried to keep it at the top of my mind.

I had more and more difficulty getting out of bed in the morning. And when I
did, I moved very slowly. However, even though my skin hurt, I did not have the
aches and pains in my large muscle groups that I experienced the year before.
Who knows why? Each of us responds differently.

I also had sharp, shooting pains in my breasts. This is a by-product for many,
I'm told. The first time was on my right side. One evening, meeting Sarah for
dinner, I was about to sit down when a sudden pain shot through my right
breast. It felt like it came from the wall of my chest and went right through the
nipple. By now, modesty about my breasts had greatly diminished, so I grabbed
that breast with both hands when the first jolt hit. I must have turned ashen
because Sarah asked me what happened. I told her—but she never experienced
that herself.

This happened again and again for the entire first year on the right side, and
sometimes during year two on both the right and the left sides. I was told by the
medical team that it was nothing to worry about. To this day, those pains still
occur on occasion. This is one of the things the doctors and nurses did not tell
me ahead of time. I wish they had.

21

Deja Vu All Over Again

○ ○
"We either make ourselves happy or miserable. The amount of work is the same."

—Collette

About three weeks after treatment began, the exhaustion started to hit. I tried to document my energy level daily, as well as whether or not my mind remained clear. On the morning of Friday, March 16, I wrote about the exhaustion in my journal. The day before, I had driven an hour to a client's office and then drove another hour at day's end to get to the radiation treatment. That was when I felt the unwelcome fatigue return. After treatment that day, the therapists starting asking how my skin was doing.

I thought, "Here it comes. The exhaustion. The skin problems. The pain." I had weird dreams at night; I slept poorly. My legs grew weak.

The fatigue depressed me, but I wanted to fight that feeling. I found books to read for escapism. I found things to look forward to—like a visit from Lucy. She timed her visit exactly when I needed a pick-me-up. Lucy is the most positive, optimistic, consistently cheerful person I know. Her visits are always the best Rx in the world. For a few Lucy-filled days, I enjoyed a much welcome reprieve from the black clouds starting to circle over my head. I needed that respite with Lucy's company over morning coffee and her buoyant demeanor throughout the day.

Sometimes a little break from routine can make all the difference. I think it helped me face the remainder of my ordeal.

Now, by Thursdays, the going got really tough for me. My whole body felt weary. My arms ached even as I drove myself home from treatment. I could barely hold them up enough to put my hands on the steering wheel of my car. Writing in my journal became increasingly difficult. I clearly understood what people meant when using the term "bone tired."

A mixed blessing was being put on hiatus by my major client, due to their decreased revenues. Although I counted on the income, I needed to stop doing anything that was non-essential. I found it difficult to focus, difficult to concentrate. My sore underarm skin made it uncomfortable to dress nicely, and the drive to the client's office seemed to take longer and longer. I was just so very weary.

In addition to the extreme exhaustion, I had increasing hot flashes (or flushes, or whatever they're called). After my first diagnosis, I stopped hormone replacement therapy which protected me from this discomfort. Later, the determination that my breast cancer was estrogen-receptive made it necessary to avoid anything that even resembled estrogen—that meant being cautious about the amount of soy and some other natural health products that I ingested. So the hot spells increased with little I could do to keep them at bay. They never got unbearable, but they were annoying and uncomfortable. I learned to dress in layers. I still seem to put on and take off articles of clothing several times each day. Later, my oncologist suggested taking Vitamin E which seems to help.

And then there were my poor breasts. I looked in the mirror and saw that the sizes were still so different from right to left. I felt very discouraged by this imbalance. My vanity had not disappeared. Eventually, they evened out, though each has its own unique surgery scar. The tiny black pindot tattoos marking each exact area of radiation will remain with me forever.

I had to force myself to do household tasks. One night while in our common laundry room, two neighbors appeared. They commented that I looked tired and asked if I felt all right. When I shared with them that I was undergoing radiation therapy, one of them told me that he had just been diagnosed with Parkinson's disease. We hugged each other.

Dread diseases. The great common denominator that can bring us closer together.

My consciousness was raised about every aspect of how I lived my life. One of those was my procrastination, a lifelong issue. I noted in my journal how much better I felt once I actually finished something that I had been avoiding and that being pleased with myself gave me a little energy boost. So, I said to myself, why not just do it (whatever "it" meant) and feel better? I try to maintain those thoughts.

I also raised my consciousness about stress, which I now think of as toxic. Avoiding stress can be very hard to do in a work world like mine that often consists of challenging deadlines, but I did my best to work ahead of the game so that the deadlines were easily met. I let my friends know that I would discourage any more anxiety than necessary in my life. Much as I used to enjoy the drama, I intended to quiet myself down.

I starting thinking that this time I should plan on just resting a bit after treatment concluded. I would take some time for myself before I continued with other things in my life.

I did a lot of internal reflection, partly because the exhaustion left me too wasted to do anything else. I thought back on the saying, "the unexamined life is not worth living." Years back I started a process of inner-examination, but it got interrupted and the time quickly filled with the busy-ness of daily life. I thought of continuing that inner quest.

I reflected on the lives of a few special women I really admired. Each of those women is independent, highly intelligent, enormously capable, and very creative. Each intentionally built the kind of life she wanted to live and the way in which she chose to live it—from her home surroundings to the way she earned income to the pursuit of her personal interests. Right and left-brainers! In each case, these women were what I deemed "complete." If romance entered their life, they felt enriched. If no significant other appeared, their lives were still wonderful. I wanted to live like that.

I looked at the things I loved. Certainly, art and beauty have always given me deep pleasure. One of my childhood dreams was to live in a pretty, color-coordinated place. I don't know why, but as a kid I thought it should be green and blue. When I grew up, I didn't even *like* green and blue, though I kept the desire to have beauty and peace around me. At long last I came to live in such a place. I have made my condo into a lovely home, and that blue and green exists through the benefit of the glorious colors in Lake Michigan, my primary view.

I love books and reading. A myriad of books interest and entice me, from novels to poetry to an assortment of non-fiction topics. I wanted a place that would hold those books and allow me a quiet and comfortable space for reading. I had that, too.

Also, I came to realize that I really like what I do for a living and the way I do it, as an independent contractor. I like an irregular lifestyle, rather than a 9-to-5 work existence. I have done both, finding each to have pros and cons, but irregularity is just more interesting to me, even though it is a peak and valley existence from both a financial and work schedule perspective. My work life is sometimes quiet, while other times I work long hours for days, evenings and weekends. Still, it affords me the possibility of taking extended weekends and vacations as I please, without having to ask permission from anyone. I like that a lot. It makes me feel free.

These reflections made me realize that, indeed, I had already created a good life for myself. Sometimes we just have to step back and see what we've got to find that we already have much of what we want…one of those forest and tree situations.

It was almost spring. I began to see the light at the end of the tunnel. I enjoyed the warmth of the bright March sun. I bought myself some daffodils. Ah, the bright yellow sunshine color. One of life's delightful treats.

Finally, I began my 10-day "countdown" till the end of treatments. I started planning the trip to Paris for my July birthday. I knew that would energize me, giving me something extra-exciting to anticipate.

By April 5th, I had just five more days to go. Once again the time came for the final five "booster" treatments—a bit of extra zapping. I knew this would really knock me out, but I also knew I was oh-so-close to the end. I felt as if I'd been holding my breath, girding myself, throughout this entire second episode.

Years back, I realized the importance of "marking" significant occasions, whether it was a promotion, or getting my MBA, or a landmark birthday, or other special life events. I wanted to mark the last day of treatment. To do so, I decided to buy a special houseplant, something big, healthy, green and beautiful. I very carefully selected exactly what I had in mind—a Peace Lily. She's been very happy at home with me and continues to honor me with the richness of her lush leaves and regularly sprouting white flowers.

22

About Fear—A Slight Digression

○ ○
"Acknowledging fear is not a cause for depression or discour-agement. Because we possess such fear, we also are potentially entitled to experience fearlessness. True fearlessness is not the reduction of fear, but going beyond fear."

—*Chogyam Trungpa Rinpoche*

My cousin, Francee, works for an incredible man, Dick Dooley, who runs Leadership Learning Forums for folks in information systems. His background included having been the CIO (Chief Information Officer—one of the top executive positions) for a huge insurance company, so Dick knows many high-level people. Over the years he came to the realization that we need to communicate better with each other, that we all can expand our thinking, and that our insides are too often overlooked—we grow through both intellectual and spiritual fulfillment.

About a week before my second surgery, Dick and I met for breakfast. He's a smart guy—easy to spot as he's 6'4" and wears a beard and a black eye patch. I already knew Dick lost his eye to cancer when he was a boy. I didn't know until that breakfast that it hit him a second time as an adult, in his stomach. I have a picture of him standing on top of a tall rock formation on the ocean with his arms spread wide to the sky. He posed for it after getting the "all clear" from his second bout. That photo is on my office wall where I see it every single day. It's my daily reminder that we beat cancer, we won!!!

Listening to Dick talk was mesmerizing for me. He is enormously well read (as evidenced in the voluminous reading list he provides to his forum participants), pretty fit (he's quite involved with tai-chi, not only for the exercise but also what he learns about control), well-traveled (he and his wife love their exotic journeys), has amazing variety in his personal contacts—and is a force, an energy source. That's the best way for me to describe him—a force! His background and mind are impressive, as is the way he chooses to share through his forums.

We met because he wanted some marketing help, but I told him I was about to have surgery and radiation, and just couldn't commit to more work right then. Dick looked surprised. "You have cancer right now? You look great!" I assured him that in spite of how I looked, I really did have cancer and wouldn't be looking or feeling so great in the near future. Of course, he knew what I meant.

I was fascinated to hear about his forums, how he brought together participants who tend to be introverts and got them to open up and share. The forums he led sounded both intellectual and spiritual and challenging, as an effective growth process should be. No wonder his participants kept coming back for more, year after year.

Dick and I kept in touch, even though I couldn't do much work for him then. A few months later Dick had a forum in the Chicago area, and invited me to participate in and observe Day One, the introductory day.

The day came, and I didn't know what to expect. To begin with, my mind was starting to get foggy from treatments. I wasn't familiar with the location of the suburban hotel and although the directions were simple, I made a wrong turn and had a longer drive than anticipated. I arrived almost on time, careful to note which specific hotel entrance I used so I'd be able to find my car when I left. These are the things you teach yourself to do when you know your mind is acting weird.

Dick welcomed me, gave me a name tag, showed me to a seat and introduced me. Most of the attendees were in the information technology field, of course, making me feel like a "ringer" among the techies. Fortunately, I can almost always find something to say to people, and once I asked them about what they had read for the forum, conversation came easily.

We listened to speakers tell about their careers, their personal lives, and their philosophies. Each had already shared their essay biographies. Essay biographies are 1-2 page narratives about the salient points of a person's life. They're not at all like resumes, or a vita, or a professional bio, which is all that I had been familiar with up to then. Although they include professional information, essay bios are far more personal. Dick insists on these. He believes that in order to work better together, we should get to know more about each other. He insisted I write one, myself, when I was invited to speak at another of his forums. It's in the beginning of this book.

The speakers were quite impressive—one was a woman who had been the CIO of Xerox, another held an equally high position elsewhere—and they talked about their work ethic and what inspired them.

Next came Dr. Carl Hammerschlag. He shared about his personal and professional life, and told us about being schooled in Western medicine before becoming involved with Native American ways. He even has a "father" who is a medicine man. Carl is a psychiatrist, an author, a healer and a wonderful speaker. He shared about his parents (holocaust survivors), education (all the way through medical school in New York), family (wife, daughters and grandkids), and about the spiritual parts of his life (from sweat lodges to more ephemeral Native American intuitive/dream topics). After that introduction, he had us in the palm of his hands. We were enthralled with his charming candor and compassion.

Carl divided us into two groups and asked each group to form a circle. He handed each of us a pencil and a sheet of the hotel's memo pads, so each piece of paper would be identical. He then told us to write down our greatest fear.

What did I get myself into?

I wrote, "I'm afraid of having cancer again." The thought of chronic cancer becoming a way of life terrified me.

We folded our papers in half, and passed them to our left—pass, pass, pass, and so on until Carl told us to stop. Then he asked us to pass them to our right, 3 times, and stop again. This way, no one knew who wrote what.

Once everyone stopped passing, he said, "Now, open the paper in your hands, and read what is written on the paper as if it were your own fear."

Wow!

The one I opened said, "My greatest fear is losing my child or grandchild."

I thought of losing my son, Adam, or my granddaughter, Angie, and the tears gushed from my eyes. I imagined the grief and knew it would be unbearable.

Suddenly, my perspective widened and my self-pity decreased. Cancer? Who cares! I've got the two people I love most in this world, and they're both healthy—nothing else is more important to me!

Others shared their greatest fears, and yes, many had written down cancer, loss of loved ones, loss of self esteem—as well as a few listing spiders and public speaking. The exercise taught us about the commonality of our fears.

A couple sat to my left. I couldn't figure out why the woman was there with her husband, an IT (information technology) guy. But then, he told us they had suffered a huge loss recently; he brought her because neither of them could yet bear to be alone. They had just lost their 10-year-old child. Death came, unexpectedly, while driving somewhere. The mother couldn't get help in time, and her dear child died. Just like that. The week before this forum she had visited the exact place of death to face the ghost. Only recently, had the couple been able to enter their child's room.

As the woman talked and the tears flowed, I put my arm around her, touching and comforting a total stranger.

One man lost his child the year before and didn't exactly know why he even came to the group this time, until he met the couple who had just lost their child. Then he knew—there was someone he needed to help. He assured them that even though they were going through a horrible time, they would get through it and go on, as he did.

When I talked about enduring my second bout with breast cancer, that woman on my left patted my shoulder, and returned the support I had just given her. We weren't strangers anymore.

This is what can happen if we can truly open up with each other—even though the tears may come, even though it might be uncomfortable at first. Once we share the fears we carry inside, our burden, our darkness becomes lighter. And we find we are not so different from one another, after all.

23

The Big Celebration

○ ○
"In the middle of difficulty lies opportunity."

—*Albert Einstein*

I planned a celebratory lunch the week after treatment ended, on Friday-the-13th (a lucky day for me). The friend with whom I celebrated became a new client almost immediately. The work that came out of that lunch date would totally occupy my mind and time for the next few months. Perfect.

Fortunately, my client allowed me my recuperation period before I had to jump in on her project with both feet. How lucky can a girl get?

Life is full of ups and downs. Shortly after my treatment ended, my mother became even more debilitated. She had been hospitalized and didn't bounce back after she came home that spring. It pained me to see her getting weaker and weaker, and to realize that her wonderful energy and zest for life would never come back the way it always had in the past.

Although I wanted my own freedom after what I had just been through, I knew this would probably be my mother's last year on earth. I promised myself to be more patient, more attentive and tried to keep my sometimes too-sharp retorts to myself. It hurt to watch her health and strength decline. She became more and more dependent on her care-giver and on me. I was her only child, after all, and she wanted as much of me as I could give her. How sad to see this little lady who adored dance now walk so slowly, reliant on the aid of a walker. She taught ballet and ballroom dance as a younger woman, and after she got a desk job, she became an international folk dancer to keep her feet moving. No dancing for mom any more. She watched her last few friends die off that year, until succumbing herself the following March. That last year with her went much too quickly.

Also, J had moved on. I didn't know if I wanted to remain in touch with him any more, but our relationship had given me so much that I found it difficult to cut it off completely. The decision to stop communicating was mine, but it tore me up. I didn't know what to do.

A chapter ends. Another begins.

Having gone through two bouts of cancer, I believed that I had a special chance at "getting things right" now for me. The indecision I felt about J at this time was all too familiar; I had been there before with prior relationships. This time, I could no longer put off facing my inner confusion and pain. The oriental sign for crisis combines the words for danger and opportunity—exactly the point I was at in my life. I did not want to blow what could be an opportunity for me.

It was time to concentrate on my inner self.

I needed help sorting out my emotions. I picked up the phone, called my former therapist, Maureen, and asked if I could come back. Yes, she had an opening. We embarked on what became an incredibly intense period of exploration for me. This time I promised myself I'd back off from nothing. This time I was determined to face my own ghosts. This time I worked hard, really hard. When I occasionally collapsed into sobbing, Maureen would ask if I'd want to stop. I never did. I insisted we continue. I knew I had to get through this process. I think it is the single best thing I've ever done for myself.

In perhaps an odd way, I realized that if it hadn't been for my deep feelings for J and the troubles we had, I might not have taken that step. This man who brought me such joy at one time, pain at another, also brought me towards finding my own path. There are no coincidences. He said to me, when talking about my return to therapy, "If you face the pain now, you'll never have to face it again." I'll never forget that. Again, wise counsel.

I decided I wanted to make a point of thanking all the many women who helped me in so many, many ways with their love, support, and encouragement. I invited them to a "healthy women" party in my home. We ate delicious, healthful food most of which I made myself because I wanted to DO something for these wonderful ladies. Sarah busied herself in the kitchen making appetizers. Another friend gave a talk on nutrition. Sandy brought some evil desserts. We broke out the wine, enjoyed the food, and laughed and laughed. A great time for the great women in my life!

Then I got my head totally into going to Paris for my birthday in July.

I asked my mom, only half-jokingly, to promise to stay as healthy as she could for the week I'd be gone. I even rented an international cell phone so she could phone me at any time. That gave us both some comfort, knowing we could easily remain in touch that week. She did just fine—and so did I!

Paris was grand, the highlight being my dinner party on Bastille Day. The guest list snowballed so that a dozen of us from America, Marseille, Paris, Germany and Amsterdam converged on my behalf for the celebration. It was a remarkable evening.

I looked around the table at one point, at these dear people, and felt that Kathleen knew we were all together that night, almost a year since she died. She had been a French scholar, studied in Paris, and would have loved the evening. I thought of her as I looked at her husband Steve, their pregnant daughter and son-in-law, and as I looked at Juliet, Steve's assistant, who had given us the updates on Kathleen's status, and at Nina who had driven with me to visit Kathleen the last time, and I thought, "Kathleen knows we're all here, she is smiling on us tonight. I'll bet she's even wishing me a happy birthday!" The only sad spot was that she couldn't join us.

Of course, I didn't care a bit about my age. Health is the biggest cause celebre there is!

Coda

The following spring, Sarah and I attended the closing ceremonies of the Avon 3-day Walk for Breast Cancer. Two friends walked 60 miles carrying my name, which was a great honor for me. I promised to cheer them on at the finish line. One of them, Lori, was a survivor herself. I went into the survivor tent area to look for her. I saw a sea of pink shirts, but found Lori and the other survivors on her team. It thrilled me to see my name imprinted on their team shirts. When I asked how many were on Tamixofen and how they were doing, the reaction was, "Ten pounds…twelve pounds…fifteen pounds!" as if they were proud of it. And why shouldn't they be? They survived! We may have been chubby, but we were alive!

My friend Shelly wore my name, too. He never had cancer. His life-altering event was walking away from a car accident when all others involved died. That made him brutally aware of priorities and perspective and the hierarchy of what we now deem "important," just as cancer had done for me.

Many months after I returned to health, my sweet friend Juliet became pregnant with twins. She and her husband Mark wanted children very much, but she had a troubled and unnerving pregnancy. I prayed for those babies and to make sure they were in good hands, I gave Juliet my angel to watch over her and her unborn children. I am happy to report that Annie worked her wonders. Sofia and William were born small but healthy, and are lovely babes.

Now my little Annie Angel has moved on again, this time to watch over another friend with advanced colon cancer. She's a busy little angel, but she does her job very, very well, as angels do.

24

What I Learned

"When you come to the edge
Of all the light you know,
And are about to step off
Into the darkness of the unknown,
Faith is knowing one of two things will happen:
There will be something solid to stand on,
Or you will be taught how to fly."

—Unknown

I have learned more and more about the yin and yang of life. Out of sadness and pain can eventually come joy—and spots of sadness may reside with pleasure. Nothing is totally one way or another. This is as it should be. That is part of our balance.

I have learned that being open with others, sharing, paves the paths between us. I have learned how important it is to be clear with those I care about. And that it can be liberating for both of us.

I have learned that some people live and others die and we'll never know why. It is what it is. It has nothing to do with fairness.

I have learned that, for me, it is never bad to love—no matter the outcome.

I have become and continue to be increasingly grateful for all the good things in my life—of which there are many. I choose to dwell on those, rather than on the bad stuff.

I have learned that you can depend on the universe to never let you down. It will provide you with what you need at the time.

I have learned that it's wonderful to believe in angels. And that they will be wonderful to you.

I've learned that we define our lives by the choices we make. I could have entered these difficult times kicking and screaming. Instead, I chose to learn from them and to share with you. I pray it's helpful to someone.

The American Cancer Society's booklet "After Breast Cancer Treatment" says:

"Everyone needs to develop their own way to live after breast cancer. More than one million women have done it—and you can, too"

APPENDIX

HELPFUL TIPS

TIPS FOR THE PERSON WITH CANCER:

1. **You are never really alone during radiation**. The first time you go in the room for treatment can be intimidating…you're one little person in a big room under a huge machine, and everybody leaves the room after you're in position. Don't worry—your radiation team is right there. They can hear you, they can see you, and they'll be right back. Really! (And don't forget, no matter where you are, your angels will never leave you—not even for a moment.)

2. **Ask your questions**. Your radiation team, most likely, will be composed of young angels who've seen more than most folks ever will. Each patient is special to them. You, too! Feel free to ask them about anything related to treatment—they've seen and heard it all.

3. **Adjust your life, for now**. This treatment thing is temporary, go along with it. The first time around I tried to fight it and keep my life as before; consequently, I put myself through a lot more than necessary. The second time, I lightened my work load, told my clients what was happening, let my family know I was planning on taking things easier, and then took time off from everything the last week of treatment and the following couple of weeks. Much easier.

4. **Yes, you'll be tired. Plan on it**. The effects of radiation are cumulative. I felt just fine most Sundays, Mondays, Tuesdays, and even up to Wednesdays. By Thursday, I felt more tired…Friday and Saturday make no (or just easy) plans…nap, rest, go with the flow. Sunday nights, I was okay again, at least for about the first four weeks. Then I got more and more tired, and by the last week of treatment, I was totally pooped!

5. **Be patient**, healing takes time. I did not really feel like myself again (I'm a pretty high energy person) until about 3-4 weeks after treatment ended. I jokingly (but not really) said it took as long to recuperate from radiation as it did to go through it.

6. **Avoid big decisions, signing contracts, and so on if you can**. If not, have someone you trust check your work. Your brain may feel "foggy." I did some really stupid things the first time around without realizing my head just wasn't functioning normally, not as sharp nor clear as usual. I have talked with many people who have had various serious illnesses and most agree that "cloudy brain" can be a real challenge. The trouble is, you may not know it's happened to you until you look back.

7. **STRETCH**. You may have aches and pains that could make you feel older than you are. The first time around I started hurting when I got up in the morning. My large muscle groups (hips, upper thighs, lower back) made me feel that I was aging at a rapidly increased rate. This did not happen the second time around. One reason may be that I tried to exercise more regularly—walk, treadmill, yoga, and s-t-r-e-t-c-h. Be gentle, but do it regularly.

8. **Get good books**. I'm a reader, and books have been my salvation in many ways. They became especially important to me during both rounds of treatment. First, to read while waiting your turn (there are all too many of us experiencing cancer and needing treatment, hence the time waiting) as well as reading while resting. I continue to pass on good book tips to others I know going through treatment. My favorites during this time were engrossing novels, those "Oprah" books and other bestsellers. The books helped me escape into someone else's life, a mini-vacation from my own.

9. **Follow instructions**. Once, I "cheated" and shaved my underarms which is not allowed, but I just couldn't stand not doing it. Big mistake. It hurt a lot and became ultra-sensitive to radiation burn. Also, you don't want to take the least little chance of nicks which can lead to infection. An electric razor is allowed, but I didn't have one at the time. Often the hair stops growing when under radiation, so it's not a major problem.

10. **Use special skin care cream early in the treatment process**. Radiation can be tough on your skin (don't worry, most of it will get back to normal). The first time, when my skin got "sunburned" I put on special cream. I had so

much discomfort, itching and tenderness that I carried the cream with me all the time so that even if I was in a restaurant or a meeting, I could go into the ladies' room and apply the stuff. The second time, I learned to start application much earlier during the treatment process. After the first week, I applied the cream immediately after treatment, while in the dressing room. Trust me, this can make a difference! Since few have had to go through treatment twice as I did, even the radiation team didn't realize how helpful this could be until I reported my success. I had something to compare that others didn't. I still had some problems the second time, but nothing as bad as the prior year. Ask your radiation team about the special care cream, even if they tell you that you don't yet need it. Start applying it early in the process.

11. **Clothing**. Be comfortable. As treatment progresses, it may get harder to wear a bra. I didn't wear one at all around the house, but as I'm well-endowed (thankfully, that is still the case), I had to wear something when going out. I got soft camisoles (pretty, too!) and tank tops with built-in shelf bras. I went to the discount stores so this didn't cost much—thanks to tips from other ladies in the waiting room.

12. **Use the waiting room to share**. Formerly, I wouldn't have shared personal stuff with a bunch of strangers. But everyone there is sort of a "sister' (or "brother," as the case may be). You're all fighting cancer and undergoing radiation therapy—quite a bond. I got some really good tips on how to handle things from other folks including the importance of stretching, encouragement for light exercise (walking), books to read, how to bathe easier without disrupting the affected area, how to go bra-less and be undetected, types of bra-substitutes (camisoles) and where to get them inexpensively, how to re-organize your day to get more rest, encouragement on asking for help, and most importantly, how to connect with other people just as interested in talking about the cancer thing as you are.

13. **Raise your consciousness in the cancer treatment waiting room**—it's a great equalizer. You'll see all kinds, each with a bond to you. Every color, every walk of life, every age—some without hair due to chemo or with a wig/hat or missing a breast and not wearing a prosthesis. I found it comforting that here we could each just be whoever we were…some dressed for business, some bra-less and casual, some tired, some upbeat, some accompanied by their children or grandchildren…but each of us fighting the same good battle!

14. **Read the brochures**. Some will be on how to care for yourself, others will be about cancer support groups. Familiarize yourself with what's available to you. That's how I found out about Gilda's Club. It's also how, a year later, I found out about Hospice care during my mother's last hospital stay. That organization is another place comprised of a full staff of angels!

15. **Keep a journal**. I didn't do this till the second time around and wish I had for the first time. You may be amazed at the profound insights and events that can happen during this experience. And if not profound, at least it can be very helpful. I kept inspirational e-mails and cards in my journal, so that when I started feeling down, I could just open the book and read them any time of the day or night. It helped a lot.

16. **Keep fresh flowers around**. I was blessed (my granddaughter, Samantha, keeps telling me I'm not "lucky," but rather that I'm "blessed"—and she's right!) with frequent flower deliveries from friends and family. There is nothing like beautiful blooms to keep your spirits up.

17. **Allow your friends to help**. I've always been so independent, it's probably actually kept people away from helping. Many friends came forward with offers, most of which I politely ignored the first time. Not so my second time around when I admitted I needed and wanted their help, and allowed myself to ask for it.

18. **It's not "over" till it's over (per the famous Yogi Berra!)**. The first time, I expected to be back to my old self the Monday following the last Friday of treatment. HAH! It took me weeks to get my energy up to its regular level. The next time around, I prepared for that in two ways. First, I did practically no work the last week of treatment, just went to movies (to stay awake) and rested and read…and continued being a sloth for another week or two. Second, after treatment I increased my work load very gradually to the longer hours I'm used to maintaining. Much smarter.

19. **Treat yourself**. I love to travel, something I couldn't do during the period of radiation treatments. The first thing I did upon completion of therapy each time was plan a special, celebratory trip.

20. **Get involved**. Join some of the walks for cancer, like the Susan G. Komen events, or the Avon walk, or the American Cancer Society, or any of the many other events supporting cancer, even if you just volunteer. Take

advantage of what's out there. If there's a Gilda's Club nearby, check it out. Or find another cancer support group. People are there to help you—all you have to do is show up.

21. **<u>Help others</u>**. Share your experiences with them; offer to help out when you can. Unfortunately, you'll probably have friends and family affected by this horrible disease. Once you've had it yourself, others will find you especially understanding and your input will be valuable to them. Often they want to talk about it. Be there for them.

22. **<u>Keep records of your medical appointments</u>**. This can be helpful in remembering what you've been told, what you're supposed to be doing, and also, to trigger your memory when all those bills come in and you have to deal with your insurance company. My claim adjuster and I got to be on a first name basis. She helped me figure out everything, as did the hospital accounts payable department. I've heard stories from others with insurance situations that were more difficult. Protect yourself, keep notes.

TIPS ABOUT THINGS THAT HELP:

1. **Cards.** I got all kinds—inspirational, humorous, thinking of you, even special ones written for people going through daily radiation treatments. (Are there now so many of us that Hallmark recognizes this category?). I kept the cards out at first, and eventually, they made their way into my journal/scrapbook.

   One friend sent me on-going fun or pretty or unusual postcards with a "prescription" that she wrote on the back, like: "Rx—funny movies" or "Rx—enjoy some art"….

   My granddaughters, Angie and Sam, made me wonderful cards. One day they came by with their folks, expecting a mid-day meal, but I had to rest before I could do anything in the kitchen. They already knew that I had breast cancer and was undergoing treatment that made me very, very tired. I wanted them to know why I wasn't my normal, energetic self.

   While I was in bed, the girls busied themselves with the papers and crayons that I keep for them. I woke up to the very best get well cards ever made. I kept them out for weeks to cheer me.

2. **E-mails:** These constant, uplifting messages became an important part of my life. My friends know I'm impatient and don't like to belabor things, and rightly assumed I'd get tired of talking on the phone about my health all the time. So they chose to write me their inspirational messages via the Internet, which is far less invasive and which I found quite welcome. Some made me laugh, some made me cry, but each made me feel better. It's amazing to find out how many people truly care. Too often we don't know about this while we're still alive and coherent.

3. **Fresh flowers:** Oh my, did I get flowers! Especially the second time around. Everyone knew how totally bummed I was, and the beautifully colored blooms did wonders for my psyche. Also, it's always a delight to receive a phone call from the doorman that says, "You've got flowers." I had them all over my house, and they cheered me as soon as I woke each day. Nothing like beauty to make one's soul smile.

4. **Stuffed animals**: I am not one of those pink-frilled, lacy, super-feminine women. I was certainly not one who continued to collect stuffed animals or dolls past her childhood. Yet one day I opened my front door to look down and see the world's silliest and most endearing polka-dot cow with a goofy face and floppy legs. I laughed out loud. The message with it (from my dear friend and neighbor, Barb) said, "To cheer you up while you're undergoing treatment every day." That ridiculous-looking cow got herself strapped into my car in such a way that I could see her in my rear view mirror every single day I drove to the hospital for treatment.

    My cousin Francee, who understands my wacky sense of humor, sent a "bedside" lady bear. I say "lady" because she had a pink straw hat sitting jauntily on one side of her head, and a pink feather boa. Her quizzical expression was both charming and funny. Whenever someone saw her they guffawed! I propped her on the window ledge in my bedroom so she'd be the first and last thing I saw each day, assuring me of a major grin waking up and going to sleep. Silly things help.

    The next year I gave her to my ailing mother to cheer her up. That lady bear proved great medicine for mom, and gave her some major laughs right up to the end of her life. The moo cow went to my dear aunt Cookie who, due to a severe stroke, had to be in a nursing home. She got some hearty chuckles, too, which leads me to the next point:

5. **Pass the good stuff on**! When you find something that helped you that you think might help someone else, let them know. Pass it on—be it a stuffed animal or a good book or a helpful suggestion. Reach out to others. Nowadays, we call that "paying it forward"...

TIPS FOR FAMILY AND FRIENDS

1. **Ask what you might do to help**. Make some suggestions. The cancer person may just be too tired or too confused to know what to ask for. Suggest some household activities like grocery shopping, laundry, housekeeping chores (changing the linens, cleaning the house), or renting and returning videos.

2. **Offer to drive them** to and from doctor appointments, hospital stays, outpatient treatment. Even if there's a regular person doing this, offer to help out. You'll be giving the care-giving person a break and giving the cancer person a new face to see, another person to talk to.

3. **Make "food" offers**. See if going out for a meal is enticing. When it's not, bringing "treats" to eat might be helpful. Ask first about what sounds appetizing since tastes can change due to medicine or treatments. Recently I brought tapioca and rice puddings to a friend going through chemo. Just what she wanted. Comfort food. Sometimes candy is welcome. Sometimes jello or sorbet. One friend sent me a canister of wonderful assorted English muffins. What a treat it was for me to choose a special one as a morning treat.

4. **Try a movie**. Movie therapy helped me stay awake a little bit longer (at least until 8:00 p.m.) in the evenings after radiation treatment. Ask if your cancer person would like that and if so, take them to the movie. A little bit of escapism can go a long way. Leave going out for dinner afterward optional.

5. **Go for a drive to see something pretty**—a body of water, forest preserves, attractive neighborhoods, beautiful houses. This requires little effort for the passenger and gets them out of the house a bit for a change of scene.

6. **Be conscious of the fact that your cancer person may tire easily**. No matter what you plan, even if you're just visiting, they may soon need to lie down and rest. Go easy. Make sure they know that you won't be offended if they're getting tired. Tell them you understand that they might want you to leave. They need to know it's not their job to entertain you, the visitor, but instead it is your job to be helpful—whatever that might mean.

7. **Check with the cancer person first, before telling others anything**. Some people are enormously sensitive about having this disease or about sharing any details. Others, like me, felt okay about getting the word out and found it oddly therapeutic.

8. **Do not phone late at night**. Cancer patients tend to tire easily. But again, ask. Each of us is different.

9. **In fact, ask about phone calls, period**. Some people become overwhelmed by an incessantly ringing phone. I found e-mail to be far less intrusive and much easier for me to manage. It allowed me to control the interaction at the times when I had the energy to do so.

10. **Gifts are nice**. Silly stuffed animals, flowers, books of light or engrossing reading (nothing too heavy either intellectually or in weight), magazines, and even loungewear. Cards are nice, too. Find things to bring a smile or inspiration or words of encouragement.

Tips for Lovers and Significant Others:

1. **Face the facts**. Once you know the test results are positive, don't try to pooh-pooh them. The person you love has cancer. Tell them that you'll be there, every step of the way.

2. **Let the cancer person talk**, sharing fears, concerns, expectations. Encourage the dialogue. Help uncover any "mysteries" by fact-finding research,

3. **Hug a lot**. Loving human touch is vital. Cuddle. Hold. Caress. Kiss. Do all the little things even if you can't do the big stuff. Be gentle—the affected areas may still be painful, so go easy.

4. **Be especially tender in your love-making**. And keep doing it as long as it is pleasurable and comfortable for the cancer person. If the person is in too much pain or discomfort or exhaustion to find enjoyment in more intense activities—then just cuddle or hold hands.

5. **Be extra-considerate and thoughtful**. Plan ahead to be helpful (or get help) with household chores. We hate to see our homes (and laundry) getting neglected just because we just can't do what we used to do.

6. **Provide occasional surprises**. Little gifts like flowers, stuffed animals, books and special cards—yes, even if you live together. Get some new flavors of tea. Have an ice cream party for two. Or buy your love a new nightgown. Or sleep shirt. Or colorful sweats. Or an oversize T-shirt with something funny written on it. Provide something to look forward to. Keep up the cheer.

7. **Do at home things together**, like crossword puzzles, board games, renting movies. Keep visitors to a minimum unless the cancer person requests more.

8. **Keep up the loving touches**—hold hands, rub their shoulders, caress their back, give massages (sure, get carried away). Make the cancer person aware that you still find their body attractive—that the chemistry between you remains.

9. **Find things to laugh about**. Laughter does wonders. Little grins and chuckles help, too.

10. **Plan a celebration** for when the treatment ends.

11. **Be playful and flirtatious**. Remind your cancer person that you find them attractive and desirable, no matter what. But don't push.

12. **Provide comfort and reassurance**. Make it clear that you cherish your loved one. As long as you can, keep your lovemaking after the diagnosis as good as before, if not better. Most importantly, just be there. Hang around. A lot!

TIPS FOR MEDICAL PROFESSIONALS:

I want to preface this with a reminder that I am writing this from the perspective of a patient. I do not presume to have any technical, medical, or scientific education.

Many, probably most, medical professionals involved with cancer patients are just wonderful. But even the most wonderful ones practice it every day and may not remember that each new patient they see is having a brand new and potentially terrifying experience.

1. **Be thoughtful**. The information you give the cancer person may be devastating, even if they look brave and practical and rational to you. Cancer is a scary word. Everything about it is frightening for most newcomers to this disease. Usually, doctors are kind when they give the dreaded diagnosis. Although the patient may seem to take it well (or not), a follow-up call from a nurse the next day or so could be extremely helpful. By then the fears and questions arise, and the cancer person might just need to talk to a knowledgeable person.

2. **Provide a glossary of terms**. Much too often busy doctors use acronyms and terminology that are totally new to the patient. Remember, we're not even used to saying something like, "my oncologist"—not the kind of doctor we'd ever choose to have in our medical repertoire, which heretofore may have included only an internist, a gynecologist, a dermatologist, etc. So, when you say "DCIS" or "clear margins," we often haven't a clue what you're talking about, but we're in too much of a confused state to say anything at the time. A day later, we're going "Whaaaat??" It would be especially nice to have a glossary of terms specifically related to our particular cancer. Most of us don't need to know everything there is to know about this disease and all its ramifications and possible treatments—just what pertains to our own situation.

3. **Give the cancer patient a "go-to" person**. I had that in Nurse Carole. She made herself available by phone, voice mail and pager for any questions before and after surgery. The doctors may be difficult to reach, so accessibility to a nurse is extremely helpful. Especially one

that's particularly knowledgeable about cancer, very understanding and very patient. Even after hours. It makes all the difference in the world.

4. **Provide easy-to-understand information**. I received a package of information from Carole with brochures and pages of explanations, as well as descriptions of what to do and what not to do. Later, a friend of mine from another hospital brought me a comic-book style rendering showing the equipment used for radiation treatment and explaining the entire process. I wish I had received that information earlier. I wanted to know everything about what was happening with my body and what was being done to it. It's the only one I've got.

5. **Be sure to review "after the fact" information**. Tell the patient what to expect AFTER surgery, and then teach them, patiently, how to care for themselves. This is especially true if the person wakes up with a drain under their arm, a colostomy bag or any other kinds of wounds requiring special attention. I wish I had known that there was a chance of fluids appearing in my breast after surgery, and more importantly, that it would be temporary. I wish I had known ahead of time that my skin was going to feel "tight" and my range of motion would be temporarily decreased and that gentle stretching would help. I wish I had known the first time how much it helped to apply special care cream after treatment even before my skin got pink. I wish I had known that my brain would get cloudy.

6. **Consider asking survivors to help with patient support**. Many of us are more than willing to reach out and help others entering the oh-so-difficult time once cancer has been diagnosed. Sarah and I would have been happy to help with any of Dr. DJ's patients if something were established for survivor support. Well, actually, it's not too late for that. We'll have to suggest that to him.Some of the biggest help comes from those who've been through it. Those who know how a soft little pillow held between the arm and the side can keep a sore underarm from being touched; those who can help you figure out how to bathe while keeping key parts dry; those who can give you tips on how to sleep with a drain in your armpit; those who've had to deal with a colostomy bag. Those are the folks who can be so very helpful to others facing these nasty experiences for the first time.

7. **Consider a "follow-up support group."** In my case, there was plentiful information around about cancer support groups and Gilda's Club, but I didn't even think to take advantage of this until the second time around. Sarah suggests establishing a slightly different kind of group for those of us already recuperated from successful surgeries who want to share and who still carry some deep-down fears of recurrences.

8. **For the receptionists.** I know you're busy and that you have a lot of paperwork and people to manage. But please, try to be pleasant to us. We might act dumb and move slow because we're still in shock from receiving a rotten diagnosis or because we're pretty sick. Treat us as you would want someone to treat you under the same situation. Remember, we really don't want to have to be in your waiting room in the first place.

SUSAN'S DO'S AND DON'TS

Susan is a survivor of a mastectomy, reconstruction and chemotherapy. Her brother-in-law is a dear friend of mine, who asked that I speak with Suzy after she was diagnosed—and scared, of course. She is married with children and is self-employed as a personal trainer and yoga instructor. We were in close touch (mostly via e-mail) from shortly after her diagnosis until she took off her wig. Susan is just fine now, thank God. In fact, when she had reconstruction, she modified both breasts, opting for slightly larger ones than the small ones she had before. She loves the way she looks now—and her new short hairdo is dynamite!

I asked her to share her own tips.

"Susan's Do's"

Give a gift of a pedicure or manicure
Give massage gift certificates
Give or refer current books
Tell them you know they are strong enough to survive this experience
Listen
Add humor to their lives
Visit them during recovery from surgery
Cook chicken noodle soup (huge pot)
E-mail often
Love their wig, no matter what
Give a foot massage

"Susan's Don'ts"

Don't give cancer books (except this one, of course)
Don't call too often
Don't give advice (unless asked for)
Don't ever comment on their wig (even if asked)
Don't tell them about an operation that's worse than theirs

Excerpts From Kathleen's Collection

Note: As far as I know, some of these were Kathleen's own words, others copied from various sources. The insights from many of them were helpful to me.

"I must be sure not to have any bad days. There is no room for energy-draining conflicts, inner or outer, and bad moods are something I simply can't afford to waste energy on."

"I grew up believing that good friends were my birthright. Now, I live in a world that treats them as an expendable luxury, despite growing indications that, far from being another burden that depletes us, friends are a vital source of energy and renewal."

"Questions which no one has a right to ask are not entitled to a truthful answer."

"Express love every day. Search for your authentic self until you find her."

"Take time to experience every moment for the unique gift it is."

"Each day is really all we can count on. Take nothing for granted. Make the most of what you get."

◆   ◆   ◆

"Don't squander precious resources: time, creative energy, emotion."

"Nurture friendship."

"You don't learn with your mouth open."

"'DNA'—Destiny, nature, aspirations…"

"Women think only perfect Norman Rockwell families can have wonderful holiday traditions. We need to continue the traditions no matter what kind of family we have. Family ritual becomes an emotional security blanket in times of stress. Traditions are the quideposts in our subconscious minds. The most powerful ones are those we can't even describe, aren't even aware of."

"The world needs dreamers who do."

"Make personal time the top priority, not the bottom."

"How we spend our days is how we spend our lives."

◆   ◆   ◆

"You cannot discover new oceans unless you have the courage to lose sight of the shore."

◆   ◆   ◆

"Home : a welcome retreat, a comfort drawer and a nest of comforts; cozy"

◆   ◆   ◆

"Too many people have lost the art of hanging out."

◆   ◆   ◆

"…how essential it is to enjoy the process of life, regarding every moment and every act as having some importance. That is how people achieve greatness in whatever they do."

◆   ◆   ◆

"Life is what you make it."
    "Don't dwell on the past, but change the present and shape the future."
    "To be healthy: eat well and exercise."
    "A mind once stretched by a new idea never regains its original dimensions."
    "Life is not a dress rehearsal—don't hold back."
    "Preserve Prime Time for real life."
    "Play hooky and luxuriate in your idleness."
    "Accept your limitations, make peace with your past."
    "Nothing in the world can take the place of persistence. Persistence and determination are omnipotent."
    "Never try to teach a pig to sing—it wastes your time and annoys the pig."
    "Never wrestle in the mud with a pig—you both get dirty and the pig loves it."

"It is people who have developed the resilience to absorb life's shocks and conflicts, without passivity, blaming, bitterness or self-destructive behaviors who are best able to enjoy life."

"The habits of brooding are rooted in the past or the future and they can rob the present moment of all harmony, beauty and joy."

"The habit of being—grateful appreciation for the good surrounding us."

"The blessing of friends: our friends are the continuous threads that help hold our lives together. Cherish your friends not in thought but in action. Friends are people who help you be more of the person you want to be."

"Enough time to pursue activities that bring you pleasure, time for family, home and soul. No 'maybe next year'"

"Leave without regret."

"Do the best you can."

"Make a difference."

"Women are the ones who 'do' Christmas, making holiday dreams come true from behind the scenes: cards, gifts, wrapping, mailing, trimming, party planning or giving."

"One of the greatest sins is the unlived life."

ATTRIBUTABLE QUOTES:

"I'd like to relax on the porch with no watch on"

>   *—Divine Secrets of the Ya-Ya Sisterhood author*

"What a wonderful life I've had. I only wish I'd realized it sooner."

>   *—Colette*

"The problem with doing nothing is not knowing when you're finished."

>   *—DeMille, Plum Island, page 1*

Albert Einstein's definition of insanity: *"Endlessly repeating the same process, hoping for a different result."*

"Home is the place where, when you go there, they have to let you in."

>   *—Robert Frost*

"Life is what happens to you while you're busy making other plans."

>   *—John Lennon*

Glossary (in alphabetical order)

The following terminology was extracted from the Web site sponsored by the Women's Information Network About Breast Cancer, www.winabc.org. I found this site particularly helpful and wish I had known about it after my first diagnosis.

Abnormal: Not normal. May be cancerous or premalignant.

Advanced (metastatic) breast cancer: A stage of cancer in which the disease has spread from the breast to other body systems by traveling through the lymphatic system or through the bloodstream.

Anesthesia: Drugs administered usually by injection or inhalation before and during surgery so that you will not feel the surgery. You may be awake (local) or asleep (general).

Anesthesiologist: A doctor who gives drugs or gases that keep you comfortable during surgery.

Antibiotic: Any of a variety of natural or synthetic substances that destroy or inhibit the growth of microorganisms. Used widely in the treatment of infections.

Antiestrogen: A substance that acts to block or modify the action of estrogen. The drug Tamoxifen is an antiestrogen.

Areola: The circular area of different pigmented skin on the breast surrounding the nipple.

Aspiration: The removal or withdrawal of fluid or tissue, by use of a needle and syringe, from a cavity to obtain cells from an area by applying suction. Cysts and lumps can sometimes be aspirated to obtain a specimen for testing.

Asymmetrical: Lack of symmetry; not matching.

Atypical cell: A mild to moderately abnormal cell.

Atypical hyperplasia: Abnormal cells that have increased in numbers; excessive growth of cells.

Axilla: The armpit.

Axillary lymph nodes: Lymph nodes draining the breast found in the armpit area.

Axillary node dissection: The surgical removal of a sampling of lymph nodes from the armpit to determine if the breast cancer has spread.

Baseline mammogram: A woman's first mammogram, used as a standard for evaluating any changes that may appear in future mammograms.

Benign: The opposite of malignant or cancerous, a benign tumor is a non-cancerous growth.

Bilateral: Pertinent to, affecting or related to two sides.

Biopsy: Excision (removal) of a piece of tissue with a syringe and needle or scalpel for microscopic examination to determine/establish a diagnosis and determine if the tissue removed is cancerous or benign.

Breast cancer: Malignant neoplasm of the breast.

Breast cancer *in situ*: Very early or noninvasive abnormal cells that are confined to the ducts or lobules in the breast. Also known as DCIS or LCIS.

Breast-conserving surgery and irradiation: A treatment option for breast cancer whereby the tumor and surrounding tissue and a sampling of axillary lymph nodes are surgically removed. The majority of the breast is preserved and the remaining breast tissue is then treated by a course of radiation therapy.

Breast self-examination (BSE): A technique that enables a woman to detect changes in her breast(s).

Calcification(s): Small deposits of calcium in breast tissue that can be detected in a mammogram. Calcification is the process by which organic tissue becomes hardened by lime salt deposits in the tissues.

Cancer: A general term for an estimated 200 different kinds of diseases characterized by the abnormal and uncontrolled growth of cells derived from normal tissues; the unregulated, disorganized proliferation of cell growth. Cancers that arise in epithelial tissues are called carcinomas.

Cancer Cell: A cell present in neoplasm having characteristics that differentiate it from normal tissue cells, such as the degree of anaplasia, irregularity in shape, indistinctness of cell outline, nuclear size, changes in the structure of nucleus and cytoplasm, increased number of mitoses (cell division) and the ability to metastasize.

Cancer grading and staging: Grading is the standardized procedure for expressing cancer cell differentiation. Cancer is graded on the differentiation of the tumor cells and the number of mitoses (cell division) present.

Staging is the extent of dissemination (distribution throughout an organ or the body) of the cancer. Staging is the process of classifying tumors, especially malignant tumors.

These procedures are useful in comparing the effectiveness of different forms of therapy.

Source: Taber's Cyclopedic Medical Dictionary, 1993, F.A. Davis Company

Chemotherapy: Systemic treatment (cytotoxic or hormonal) with drugs that reach cells throughout the body; used to kill or slow down the growth of cancer cells.

Clear margins: An area of normal tissue that surrounds cancerous tissue, as seen during examination under a microscope.

Core Biopsy: A biopsy using a small needle to cut and remove a sample of tissue from a breast lump.

Cyst: A fluid-filled mass or area in the breast.

DCIS, ductal carcinoma in situ (intraductal carcinoma): Abnormal cells that involve only the lining of a milk duct.

Diagnosis: The term specifying the name of the disease or syndrome that a person has or is believed to have.

Diagnostic mammogram: A diagnostic mammogram is used to evaluate a woman with symptoms suggestive of breast cancer found during physical examination such as a palpable lump or thickening of breast tissue or when a problem is detected in a screening mammogram, such as a shadow or spot requiring further investigation.

Drain: Tubes or suction devices inserted after a mastectomy or breast reconstruction to drain the fluids that accumulate following surgery.

Duct: A tubular structure in the breast that milk passes through to the nipple.

Ductal carcinoma in situ (DCIS): A type of breast cancer found in the breast ducts that has not become invasive. Also referred to as intraductal carcinoma.

Estrogen or progesterone receptor (ER/PR) Analysis: A test used to measure or detect the presence of estrogen or progesterone receptors in a tumor. The presence or absence of these receptors is important in determining whether or not the cancer is sensitive to estrogen and/or progesterone hormones in the body and whether or not cytotoxic or hormonal therapy will be used.

Excise: To cut or remove surgically.

Excisional biopsy: The surgical removal of the entire lump.

Fine needle aspiration (FNA): A biopsy using a thin needle to remove fluid from a cyst or a group of cells from a solid lump.

Glands: Lymph nodes.

Guided imagery: Imagining yourself in a story told by someone else. A flow of thoughts that you can see, hear, feel, smell or taste in your imagination.

Gynecologist: A doctor who specializes in the care and treatment of women's reproductive systems.

Hormones: Chemical substances produced in one part of the body and carried in the blood to another part of the body, where it has specific effects.

Hormone receptor assay: A diagnostic test to determine if a breast cancer's growth is influenced by hormones and/or can be treated with hormone therapy.

Hormone therapy: Treatment of cancer to block the ability of hormones to interact with cancer cells. Tamoxifen is an example of a drug used in hormone therapy.

Incisional biopsy: The surgical removal of a portion of an abnormal area of tissue or lump.

Infiltrating (invasive) cancer: Cancer that has spread outside of its site of origin to infiltrate and grow in surrounding tissue.

In situ cancer: Very early or noninvasive growths confined to the ducts or lobules in the breast. In situ means "in the site of." When used to describe a type of cancer, in situ refers to tumors that have not grown past their site of origin and have not spread into surrounding tissue.

Intravenous (IV): Within or into a vein. An intravenous line is when a needle is inserted into a vein to carry through blood products, medications or nutrients directly into the blood through a tube.

Invasive (infiltrating) cancer: Cancer that has the tendency to spread outside of its site of origin to infiltrate and grow in surrounding, healthy tissue. Invasive does not indicate that the cancer has already spread.

Irradiation: The therapeutic application of radiation to a patient to destroy or damage cancer cells. Cancer cells have a tendency to be more easily destroyed than the normal cells in surrounding tissue. Irradiation is a method of treatment for breast cancer patients, often used as an adjunctive therapy to breast-conserving surgery (lumpectomy) to minimize the risk of recurrence.

Lobular carcinoma in situ (LCIS): Abnormal cells within the lobule that do not form lumps. Lobular carcinoma in situ can serve as a marker of increased cancer risk.

Lobules: Parts of the breast capable of producing milk.

Local treatment of cancer: Treatment of the tumor only.

Localization biopsy: The use of mammography or ultrasound to locate a suspicious area that cannot be felt by hand.

Localized cancer: A cancer confined to its site of origin.

Lump: A mass of tissue.

Lumpectomy: The surgical removal of a malignant tumor along with a small margin of surrounding tissue. This surgery is usually followed by radiation therapy in the treatment of breast cancer.

Lymph: A transparent, slightly yellow fluid that carries lymphocytes, bathes the body tissues and drains into the lymphatic vessels.

Lymphatic vessels: A body-wide network of channels similar to the blood vessels that transport lymph to the immune organs and into the bloodstream.

Lymph nodes: Structures in the lymphatic system that act as filters to keep particulate matter like bacteria from entering the bloodstream. They may also stop cancer cells and help the body's immune system. Lymph nodes are small bean-shaped organs of the immune system that vary in size from a pinhead to the size of an olive and may occur singly or in groups. Lymph nodes are distributed widely throughout the body and linked by lymphatic vessels found in regions. The main areas in which they are found are in the neck (cervical), the armpit (axillary) and in the groin (inguinal).

Lymphedema: A condition characterized by swelling from the collection of fluid in the hand and arm after lymph nodes are blocked or removed.

Malignant: Cancerous.

Mammogram: A low-dose breast x-ray that details the structure of breast tissue. A method of breast cancer detection.

Marker: A device or substance used to indicate or mark something. An identifying characteristic or trait that permits seemingly similar materials or disease conditions to be differentiated (distinguished).

Mastectomy: The surgical removal of the breast, usually for treatment of cancer.

Meditation: Any activity that keeps the attention pleasantly anchored in the present moment. There are two basic approaches to meditation: concentrative meditation which focuses the attention on an image, a sound (mantra) or the breath in order to quiet the mind and mindfulness meditation which involves a broader focus of attention on what is going on all around a person without the person becoming involved in thinking about or reacting to the activities with memories, thoughts, images or worries.

Microcalcification: Tiny calcifications (calcium deposits) in the breast tissue usually detected only on a mammogram. Microcalcifications are a sign of change within the breast and, if clusters are present, may be a sign of ductal carcinoma in situ.

Multidisciplinary: Refers to multiple disciplines (specialties) involved in patient care. This term implies that the various specialties (surgery, plastic surgery, radiation/radiology, oncology, etc.) are working in collaboration and interacting with one another with respect to patient care.

Needle aspiration: A diagnostic method of removing fluid or a sample of tissue from a breast tumor or cyst by use of a fine needle for microscopic examination/evaluation.

Needle biopsy: Removal of a small sample of tissue with a wide-bore needle and suction.

Needle localization: A procedure used to pinpoint a breast lump prior to a biopsy.

Oncologist: A doctor or scientist who specializes in oncology (in treating cancer). There are medical, radiation and surgical oncologists.

Oncology: The branch of medicine specializing in tumors and the study and treatment of cancer.

Palliative: Relieving/alleviating a symptom (i.e., pain) without curing the cause.

Palpable: Perceptible, especially by touch.

Pathologist: A physician who specializes in diagnosing the abnormal changes in tissues and cells and the diagnosis of disease through the study of tissues and cells.

Pathology: The study of the nature and cause of disease, which encompasses changes in structure and function.

Positive nodes: Lymph nodes that have been invaded by cancer cells.

Predisposition: The potential susceptibility to develop a particular disease or condition in the presence of specific conditions.

Primary cancer: The area where cancer begins. Primary cancer is usually named after the organ in which it starts.

Prognosis: The forecast of the expected or probable outcome of a disease and the prediction/estimate of the chance for recovery.

Radiation oncologist: A doctor who uses radiation therapy to treat cancer.

Radiation therapist: A health professional who gives radiation treatment.

Radiation therapy (radiotherapy, radiation oncology): The branch of medicine that uses ionizing radiation in the treatment of cancer.

Radiologist: A physician who specializes in diagnosing and treating disease by the use and analysis of x-ray films and other images.

Range of motion exercises: Exercises to prevent loss of motion through movement of joints (i.e., wrist, elbow, shoulder) through their available range of motion. Often recommended following breast surgery.

Receptor: In pharmacology, a cell component that joins with a drug, hormone or chemical mediator to alter the function of the cell.

Recurrence: Return of symptoms/disease after a period of dormancy, as in the return of cancer following treatment. Local recurrence refers to a tumor/cancer that has returned to the same location as the original cancer.

Risk factor(s): Factors/conditions such as those conditions in the environment, or genetic, physiological, psychological or chemical elements that are thought to predispose a person to the development of a disease.

Screening (baseline) mammogram: Screening is the process of assessing healthy people with no symptoms present in order to detect early signs of a disease. The purpose of a screening or baseline mammogram is to establish a record of healthy breast tissue appearance against which later changes in breast tissue can be compared.

Sentinel lymph node: The first lymph node(s) to which cancer cells spread after leaving the area of the primary tumor. Presence of cancer cells in this node alerts the doctor that the tumor has spread to the lymphatic system.

Side effects: Unintentional or undesirable secondary effect of treatment.

Staging: Classification system, using TNM system (tumor, node, metastasis) to determine extent of cancer and treatment.

Stereotactic needle biopsy: Procedure that pinpoints area of concern with a double-view mammogram and, by computer, guides a fine or large-core needle for removal of tissue sample.

Surgeon or surgical oncologist: A doctor who performs biopsies and other surgical procedures such as removing a lump or a breast.

Tamoxifen: Estrogen blocker used in treating breast cancer.

Therapy: Treatment.

Tumor: An abnormal growth of tissue. Tumors may either be benign (not cancer) or malignant (cancer).

Tumor markers: Proteins, antigens, genes and ectopically produced hormones that are released from the tumor into the blood or produced by normal tissue in response to the tumor.

Tumor, Node, Metastasis System (TNM): Cancer classification system using the size of the tumor, number of lymph nodes involved as well as spread of cancer to other organs.

Two-step procedure: Biopsy and additional surgery done in two stages, usually a week or more apart.

Visualization: Use of imagery and visual pictures to help reduce stress and to promote healing.

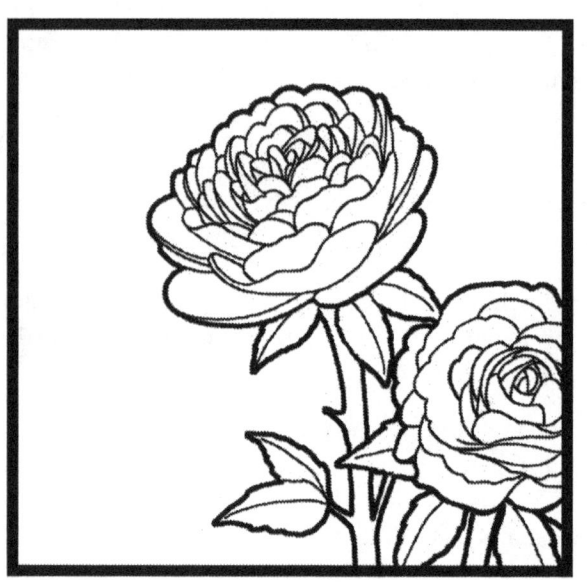

0-595-28168-0

www.ingramcontent.com/pod-product-compliance
Lightning Source LLC
Chambersburg PA
CBHW061311280526
45784CB00002B/959